Praise for *Why We Get Sick*

"If one reads headlines about the health of folks in developed nations, it's a depressing read. Heart disease, diabetes, neurodegeneration such as Parkinson's and Alzheimer's . . . all increasing. We know more about these diseases than ever before, yet we seem virtually powerless to do anything about them. But what if, instead of all these conditions and disease being separate and unconnected, one physiological state— elevated insulin levels—was the driver of all this suffering? In *Why We Get Sick*, Benjamin Bikman unpacks the root cause of modern diseases and provides a concise road map to help you regain or maintain your health."

> —*Robb Wolf,* New York Times *and*
> Wall Street Journal *bestselling author*

"This book is a unique, rigorous contribution to understanding insulin resistance as an underlying cause of chronic disease and aging. Well written and highly accessible, Dr. Bikman has written a book for both scientists and the average reader who seeks a path back to good health."

> —*Nina Teicholz, science journalist and* New York Times
> *bestselling author of* The Big Fat Surprise

"It's time to make 'insulin resistance' part of the public lexicon. That so many people are unaware of this widespread condition with serious ramifications is a monumental problem, and it's one that *Why We Get Sick* sets out to solve."

> —*Dr. Aseem Malhotra, cardiologist and*
> *professor of evidence-based medicine*

"Thoroughly researched and extensively documented, *Why We Get Sick* is a comprehensive and indispensable primer on insulin resistance and how it affects virtually every system in the body. Dr. Bikman presents not only an easy-to-understand guide to how and why insulin resistance develops, but a treatment handbook as well. If you want to understand the underlying basis for most of the diseases plaguing the industrialized world right now and how to remedy them, this is the book for you. Highly recommended!"

"Insulin resistance underpins nearly every single chronic disease that we struggle with today and ultimately costs us countless billions of dollars in health-care spending, as well as an untold amount of human suffering. Professor Ben Bikman masterfully lays out the role of insulin resistance in disease, how it affects our bodies, and, most important, how to fix it! Scientific references back every statement that he makes and, despite being science focused, it is very accessible for all audiences and a thoroughly enjoyable read!"

"Professor Bikman's sweeping summary of the science of human metabolism makes the ironclad case for insulin resistance as Public Health Enemy #1. Whether the reader is interested in losing excess body fat, optimizing brain function, preventing heart disease, reducing cancer risk, or improving fertility—this expert curation of the research leaves no stone unturned. There are very few authors with the expertise and ability to connect the data dots in a way that health-care professionals, researchers, and the science-savvy public can trust. This meticulously referenced book will undoubtedly serve as a valuable resource for years to come."

WHY
WE GET
SICK

WHY
WE GET
SICK

The Hidden Epidemic at the Root
of Most Chronic Disease—and How to Fight It

Benjamin Bikman, PhD

BenBella Books, Inc.
Dallas, TX

BenBella Books, Inc.
10440 N. Central Expressway, Suite 800
Dallas, TX 75231
www.benbellabooks.com
Send feedback to feedback@benbellabooks.com

BenBella is a federally registered trademark.

Printed in the United States of America
10 9 8 7 6 5 4 3 2 1

Library of Congress Control Number: 2019059826
ISBN 9781948836982 (hardcover)
ISBN 9781950665174 (ebook)

Editing by Claire Schulz
Copyediting by James Fraleigh
Proofreading by Karen O'Brien and Amy Zarkos
Indexing by WordCo Indexing Services, Inc.
Text design by Publishers' Design & Production Services, Inc.
Text composition by Aaron Edmiston
Cover design by Oceana Garceau
Cover image © iStock / nadla
Printed by Lake Book Manufacturing

Distributed to the trade by Two Rivers Distribution, an Ingram brand
www.tworiversdistribution.com

Special discounts for bulk sales are available.
Please contact bulkorders@benbellabooks.com.

For Cheryl, Samara, Elizabeth, and Asher

CONTENTS

FOREWORD

MEDICAL SCIENCE has advanced considerably in the last century. In 1900, the top three killers were lung infections (pneumonia or influenza), tuberculosis, and gastrointestinal infections. So, if you asked the question in 1900, "Why do we get sick?" the answer, overwhelmingly, would be "infectious diseases." But this is no longer true. With improved sanitation, personal hygiene, and miraculous medications such as antibiotics and antivirals, infections no longer kill as many Americans.

Today, if we ask the question, "Why do we get sick?" we get a very different answer. The top two causes of death, as well as five of the top seven causes (heart disease, cancer, cerebrovascular disease, Alzheimer's disease, and diabetes), are related to chronic metabolic diseases.[1] Over the past few decades, all these conditions have been on the rise. But why? You're about to learn that a lot of it comes down to one root cause: insulin resistance and hyperinsulinemia (meaning too much insulin in the blood). But, wait—isn't that actually two root causes? No, they are the same thing, like two sides of the same coin, differing only in the way you look at it.

As a nephrologist, I specialize in kidney disease, and the most common cause of kidney disease is type 2 diabetes. In only 30 years, the number of people with diagnosed diabetes has quadrupled, and I've seen its disastrous effects firsthand. It's not just about kidney disease. Patients with type 2 diabetes are also at hugely increased risk of heart disease, stroke, cancer, blindness, nerve damage, amputation, and chronic infections.

All chronic diseases involve a number of different causes and factors, but we know that type 2 diabetes, the prototypical state of hyperinsulinemia and insulin resistance, is one of the biggest. And our failure to understand the root causes of diabetes means that our approach to diagnosing and treating it is all wrong. Patients get diagnosed with type 2 diabetes only when their blood glucose gets out of control. But the causes of this disease—excess body weight and increasing resistance to insulin—are present long before the diagnosis is made. As Dr. Benjamin Bikman explains in *Why We Get Sick*, we need to be looking at insulin; insulin resistance is a precursor to diabetes and is implicated in many other conditions. *Why We Get Sick* connects the dots between insulin resistance and problems of the head, heart, blood vessels, internal organs, and more, to create a startling picture of why chronic conditions are on the rise and what we can do about it. And this is where Ben's expertise as a professor and scientist (and author) really shines.

I first met Dr. Ben Bikman when we were both presenting at an international nutrition conference. I was discussing the clinical benefits of intermittent fasting on obesity and type 2 diabetes, both primarily diseases of hyperinsulinemia. Ben was presenting the molecular processes underlying insulin and its influence on health and disease. What I was seeing clinically, Ben was studying scientifically in his lab, and I was immediately impressed with how he explained many of the metabolic benefits I was seeing in my patients. Ben is both knowledgeable and articulate, a rare combination. He obviously understands insulin inside and out, but he's also able to transmit that knowledge to a lay audience, making it simple and understandable. I've since listened to several more of Ben's lectures and always come away impressed, having learned something new. Ben has a laser-quick mind, able to cut right to the heart of the problem without getting lost in other distractions. He now makes his knowledge available in this new book, *Why We Get Sick*.

Like Ben, I am an author, and in my previous books, I explored what makes us gain weight and how this connects with type 2 diabetes. *The Obesity Code* and *The Diabetes Code* highlighted the relevance of insulin and what happens when we have too much. In *Why We Get Sick*, Ben tackles a similar question, but on a broader scale, by identifying insulin as what leads us to develop chronic disease. The scope is enormous—but, surprisingly, so much of it comes back to what Ben calls "a humble hormone from the pancreas." Ben has collected an incredible amount of research to paint a clear picture of this hormone and its far-reaching effects throughout our bodies—when we're in good health and when we're getting sick.

Insulin emerges as a key player in many of the diseases that, unfortunately, are becoming remarkably common, from migraine headaches to fatty liver disease, high blood pressure, and dementia. Ben reveals the scientific studies linking these seemingly distinct health problems (and more) to insulin resistance. And, like so many other health disorders, this one is all too common; a recent study suggests that as many as 85% of American adults may be insulin resistant, and many other countries are likely at similar levels or worse.[2]

Why We Get Sick does much more than sound the alarm bells about this prominent yet little-known condition. Although its consequences are dire if left untreated, insulin resistance doesn't have to be a life sentence. There are simple, science-based approaches to reverse the condition or prevent it from developing. And none of these approaches involve taking more medications, having more surgery, or receiving more medical implants. Instead, the solution lies in our diet and lifestyles.

This is not just another admonition to eat fewer calories and start jogging. Ben takes us far beyond this failed "eat less, move more" calorie-based approach to the more nuanced, physiological insulin-based perspective. Ben's sound strategy focuses on easy but powerful diet and lifestyle changes to bring insulin back to healthy levels. While some of the evidence Ben shares supports conventional medical practice, he reveals that insulin resistance is largely a product of our daily choices; thus, our lifestyle is both the culprit and, with some helpful and unconventional insight, the cure.

Yes, insulin resistance may be "the epidemic you may have never heard of." But if we're to curb our rising rates of obesity, diabetes, Alzheimer's, heart disease, and more, it's time for a closer look at insulin . . . and to recognize that the key to good health is already in your hands.

—*Dr. Jason Fung*

INTRODUCTION

W E ARE SICK. Worldwide, we are struggling with diseases that were once very rare—and in many cases, we're losing the fight. Each year, roughly 10 million people die from cancer and almost 20 million people die from heart disease around the world. Another 50 million people globally have Alzheimer's disease, and almost a half a billion of us have diabetes.

While diseases like these are becoming increasingly common, other, less lethal conditions are also on the rise. Roughly 40% of adults worldwide are considered overweight or obese. Furthermore, almost half of men over 45 have lower-than-optimal testosterone levels, and almost 10% of women experience menstrual irregularities or infertility.

Though they may seem unrelated, all of these disorders and more do have one thing in common: to varying degrees, insulin resistance is causing the problem or making it worse. And you might have it, too. Odds are you do—a recent study hints that up to 85% of all US adults may have it,[1] along with half of all adults in Mexico, China, and India, and more than one third of adults in Europe and Canada. The problem is at least as prevalent across the Pacific Islands, North Africa, and the Middle East.

In fact, *insulin resistance is the most common health disorder worldwide*, and it affects more people—adults and children—each year than any other. And yet most people are not familiar with the term "insulin resistance," or if they are, they don't understand it. Not surprising—I'm a biomedical scientist and professor, and though I now focus on insulin resistance, I was once totally in the dark about this condition, too.

How I Became an Expert on a Disease I'd Never Heard of

If you're wondering why you haven't heard more about insulin resistance given how common it is, you aren't alone. I certainly wasn't familiar with it until my professional academic interests pulled me in that direction. Even then, I hadn't set out to study insulin resistance, but my interests quickly began to shift.

In the early 2000s, like now, obesity was receiving plenty of attention. After reading a scientific article about how fat tissue secretes hormones that flow through the blood and affect all other parts of the body, I was fascinated—and I had to learn more. My research had originally focused on how muscles adapt to exercise, but that article got me interested in how the body adapts to obesity—and why wouldn't it? The human body is amazing and determined to keep functioning even in unhealthy conditions like obesity. (Unfortunately, as you'll learn, not all adaptations are beneficial.) The more articles I read, the more the evidence suggested that as the body gains fat, it also becomes insulin resistant, or less and less responsive to the hormone's effects.

While my graduate studies began scratching at the surface of the *origins* of insulin resistance, I was still completely naïve as to how insulin resistance, in turn, causes other diseases. That awakening happened when I became a university professor.

My first teaching assignment was to instruct undergraduates about how our body systems operate when we have a disease or injury—a subject called pathophysiology. As a scientist, I'd been studying what causes insulin resistance; at the time, however, I didn't really think it was connected to chronic diseases, other than as a precursor to type 2 diabetes and a tangential link to heart disease.

Once I started putting lectures together for my classes, I played to my strengths by focusing on insulin resistance whenever I could. And that was when my eyes were opened. In particular, I remember preparing a lecture on cardiovascular disorders—the world's leading cause of death—and I was dumbfounded when I found countless scientific manuscripts highlighting the many different ways in which insulin resistance directly caused high blood pressure, high cholesterol, arterial plaques, and more. The link was more than tangential!

I began trying to find any evidence of insulin resistance in other diseases, and I learned that it was present in almost *every* chronic disease. (It was especially present in the chronic conditions that stem from a diet high in processed and artificial foods, as you will see.)

This was something I'd never really appreciated—insulin resistance causing diseases other than diabetes—and yet I was considered an expert on insulin resistance!

As embarrassed as I was by my lack of knowledge, I was equally amazed that most other scientists and physicians were just as ignorant as I had been. And if other biomedical professionals weren't aware of insulin resistance as a single cause of the most common chronic diseases, I figured that the average person would be almost completely in the dark. I wondered why insulin resistance *wasn't* more commonly discussed in health conversations. But with time, I realized that for someone to grasp the enormity of the problem, they would have to comb through thousands of scientific journals and manuscripts, understand the jargon, and be able to connect the dots. Even more difficult, they'd have to translate that research into practice. No wonder so few people recognized the threat of insulin resistance.

More recently, as the scope of the problem has become ever more obvious, I've been invited to discuss my research. I've since been able to share this message around the world, via public speaking engagements, podcast interviews, and YouTube discussions. However, no amount of speaking gives me enough time to say all I want to on the topic. That's where this book comes in.

My main goal is to demystify the science of insulin resistance, so that anyone can appreciate what it is and why it's dangerous. I want to arm you with the knowledge of how to prevent and even reverse insulin resistance, all based on sound and published evidence. And I want to teach you the steps to preventing disease through simple lifestyle changes—no prescriptions required.

The research that I rely on in this book has been performed and published by hundreds of different labs and hospitals all over the world that have studied this issue for a century. As an author and scientist, I find this history of evidence liberating—nothing I write in this book is based on my opinion, but rather published, peer-reviewed science. (So, if you find any of these conclusions inconvenient, I'm afraid you'll have to take on the primary evidence.)

How Do I Know if I Have It?

As I mentioned, many medical professionals are unaware of how common insulin resistance is, the problems it can cause, and, most importantly, how to identify it. So even if your doctor has never brought it up, you may not be out of the woods.

To get a sense of your risk level, answer these questions:

- Do you have more fat around your belly than you'd like?
- Do you have high blood pressure?
- Do you have a family history of heart disease?
- Do you have high levels of blood triglycerides?
- Do you retain water easily?
- Do you have patches of darker-colored skin or little bumps of skin ("skin tags") at your neck, armpits, or other areas?
- Do you have a family member with insulin resistance or type 2 diabetes?
- Do you have polycystic ovarian syndrome (PCOS; for women) or erectile dysfunction (for men)?

All of these questions reveal some connection to insulin resistance. If you answered "yes" to one question, you likely have insulin resistance. If you answered "yes" to any two questions (or more), you most certainly have insulin resistance. In both instances, this book is for you. Read it and learn about the most common disorder in the world, why it's so common, why you should care, and what you can do about it. It's time to look at your health differently, and you can get a clearer picture of your disease risk and address potential problems by focusing on insulin.

How to Read This Book

To take full advantage of this book, you need to remember the three reasons I wrote it:

1. to help people become familiar with insulin resistance, the world's most common health disorder;

2. to provide information on insulin resistance's link to chronic diseases, and;
3. what to do about it.

These three aims are divided across the "parts" of the book. Part I, "The Problem: What Is Insulin Resistance and Why Does It Matter?" describes insulin resistance and the many diseases and conditions that can result from it. If you're already very familiar with the connection of insulin resistance to numerous chronic diseases and you're curious about its origins instead, skip to Part II, "Causes: What Makes Us Insulin Resistant in the First Place?" If you've already learned the causes and consequences of insulin resistance and you're eager to see and understand the science underpinning the best dietary strategy to address it, start reading with Part III, "The Solution: How Can We Fight Insulin Resistance?"

Of course, for most readers, even those who *think* they know what insulin resistance is and why it matters, I'd recommend starting at the beginning; what you don't know about insulin resistance will surprise you.

Because of how many diseases are associated with insulin resistance, I've dedicated a good part of this book to exploring how it can make us very, very sick. Many of the diseases we will cover—type 2 diabetes, heart disease, Alzheimer's, and certain cancers—are serious and have no known cure. So, you may sometimes feel like you're reading a horror story. But don't despair; despite all the serious chronic diseases stemming from it, insulin resistance *can* be prevented and even reversed, and we'll explore how in great detail. While things you read here may frighten you, this book at least has a happy ending—we can fight, and when armed with science-based solutions, we can win.

PART I

The Problem

What Is Insulin Resistance and Why Does It Matter?

CHAPTER 1

What Is Insulin Resistance?

INSULIN RESISTANCE is the epidemic you may have never heard of.
Though many of us are unfamiliar with it, our unawareness belies how common it really is: half of all US adults, and roughly one in three Americans, are known to have it.[1] However, this number could be as high as 88% of adults![2]

Even more disturbing is how common it will be in the future—and don't think the problem is just local. When we look at worldwide trends, it gets even grimmer: 80% of all individuals with insulin resistance live in developing countries, and, as in America, half of all adults in China and India are insulin resistant. Still, this isn't a new trend. According to the International Diabetes Federation, the number of cases of insulin resistance worldwide has doubled in the past three decades and will likely double again in less than two more.

Insulin resistance was once a disease of affluence (what I like to call a "plague of prosperity"), or a condition that largely affected only well-off older people. Recently, however, that has all changed—there are documented reports of insulin-resistant four-year-olds (and up to 10% of North American children have it[3]). And low-income countries have passed high-income countries in terms of total number of people with the condition.[4]

To top it all off, the overwhelming majority of people with insulin resistance *don't know they have it* and have never heard of it! So when it comes to combating rising global rates of this disease, we have an additional barrier: getting people to understand it in the first place.

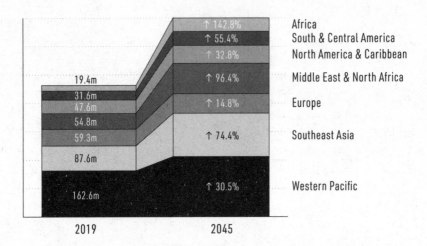

Current and projected cases of diabetes by region (in millions)
Data source: International Diabetes Federation[5]

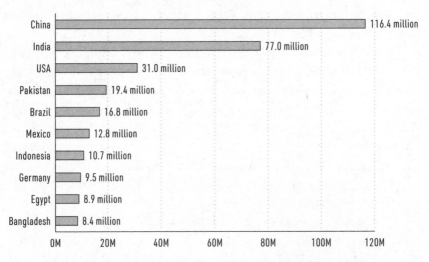

Top 10 countries by number of adults with diabetes in 2019
Data Source: International Diabetes Federation[6]

Introducing Insulin

Before we can understand insulin resistance, we need to lay the groundwork by discussing insulin itself. Many people only think of insulin as a medication for people with diabetes. Insulin is actually a hormone that we naturally produce in our bodies (unless we have type 1 diabetes—more on that later).

Like most hormones, insulin is a protein that is manufactured in one part of the body, moves through our blood, and affects other parts of the body. In insulin's case, it's made in the pancreas, a small organ tucked beneath the stomach. Insulin's most famous role is regulating our blood glucose levels. When we eat food that increases blood glucose, the pancreas releases insulin, which then "opens the doors" to escort glucose from the blood to various parts of the body, such as the brain, heart, muscles, and fat tissue. And yet, far beyond regulating our blood glucose, insulin has an effect on every cell in every tissue of the body—a pretty big audience! This is almost unheard of among hormones; usually they affect only one or perhaps a few organs, but not insulin—its heavy hand touches every cell.

The specific effect of insulin depends on the cell. For example, when insulin binds to a liver cell, the liver cell makes fat (among other things); when insulin binds to a muscle cell, the muscle cell makes new proteins (among other things). From the brain to the toes, insulin regulates how a cell uses energy, changes its size, influences production of other hormones, and even determines whether cells live or die. Common among all of its effects is insulin's ability to have the cell make bigger things out of smaller things, a process known as anabolism. Insulin is an anabolic hormone.

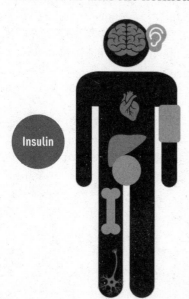

Brain: Glucose use for energy, neuron growth

Ears: Glucose use for energy, hearing

Heart: Energy use, heart size, lowers blood pressure

Muscle: Energy use, muscle protein production, size

Fat: Glucose conversion to fat, fat storage, growth

Liver: Glucose storage, fat production

Testicles/Ovaries: Normal sex hormone production

Bone: Energy use, growth

Nerves: Glucose use for energy, growth

Insulin's many functions

Clearly, insulin is important—when it works! The problem, and much of the point of this book, is when insulin isn't working correctly, a state defined as insulin resistance.

Defining Insulin Resistance

At its simplest, insulin resistance is a reduced response to the hormone insulin. When a cell stops responding to insulin, which can be caused by various conditions (covered later), it becomes insulin resistant. Ultimately, as more cells throughout the body become insulin resistant, the *body* is considered insulin resistant.

In this state, certain cells need more than normal amounts of insulin to get the same response as before. Thus, the key feature of insulin resistance is that blood levels of insulin are higher than they used to be, and the insulin often doesn't work as well.

"BLOOD GLUCOSE" OR "BLOOD SUGAR"?

The term "blood sugar" is vague and misleading, but technically accurate as all simple carbohydrates can be termed "sugars." "Sugar" has commonly come to mean sucrose (that is, table sugar and high-fructose corn syrup), a compound made from joined glucose and fructose molecules. But this isn't the sugar we mean when we talk about "blood sugar." The more accurate term is glucose, the invariable final form of the carbohydrates we consume once they are digested.

As mentioned, one of insulin's main roles is regulating our blood glucose. Because sustained high glucose levels are dangerous, even potentially lethal, our bodies need insulin to usher the glucose from the blood, effectively lowering blood glucose back to normal. But what about glucose control with insulin resistance? As insulin resistance settles in, this process becomes compromised, which can lead to high blood glucose levels, or "hyperglycemia"—the universal sign of diabetes. But we're getting ahead of ourselves; insulin resistance can be present long before a person develops type 2 diabetes. (For a description of the difference between diabetes types 1 and 2, see the next section.)

Insulin is almost always considered in the context of glucose, which isn't entirely fair considering the hundreds (thousands?) of things insulin does throughout the body. Nevertheless, in a healthy body, if blood glucose is normal, insulin is usually normal. However, with insulin resistance, insulin levels are *higher* than expected relative to glucose. In the "story" of insulin resistance and diabetes, we've been treating glucose as the main character, but it's really the sidekick. That is, glucose is the typical blood marker we use to diagnose and monitor diabetes, but we should really be paying attention to insulin levels first.

So why the backward priority? Well, we can likely blame the glucose-centric paradigm of insulin resistance and type 2 diabetes on history and science.

Why Too Many Focus on Glucose, but Not Insulin

Historically, because it is a cause of type 2 diabetes, insulin resistance has been lumped into the diabetes mellitus family of diseases.

The first recorded evidence of this family comes from ancient Egypt over 3,000 years ago, through a medical papyrus noting that people with a particular condition experienced "too great emptying of the urine." Some time after, physicians in India observed that certain individuals produced urine that attracted insects like honey. (In fact, that symptom would inspire part of the name for the disease: "mellitus" is Latin for honey-sweet.)

Hundreds of years later, in Greece, the excessive urine associated with the disease elicited the name *diabete*, which means "to pass through," further emphasizing the remarkable amount of urine patients were producing. All of these observations also came with one common finding: in each case, the excessive urine production was accompanied with weight loss. In fact, though it seems amusing now, early theories were that the flesh was melting into urine.

These early physicians, and those that came later, were describing type 1 diabetes mellitus. It wasn't until the fifth century that Indian physicians noted two distinct types of this disease, one associated with a young age and losing weight (which modern physicians would come to call type 1), the other with older age and excess body weight (type 2). Nonetheless, both were identified by the excess amount of glucose-loaded urine. In the absence of savvier techniques, this under-standably lead to the disease being defined by glucose, which was caus-ing the common, main observable symptom (polyuria—the technical term for producing too much pee).

However, in doing so, we ignored the other, more relevant half of the problem—insulin. And while diabetes types 1 and 2 share the symptom of excess glucose, they diverge completely when it comes to insulin. Whereas type 1 diabetes is caused by having too little insulin (or none), type 2 is caused by having too much.

This "too much insulin" is insulin resistance, and because of its association with type 2 diabetes, it became wrapped up in the glucose-centric perspective as well.

MODY: LOOKS LIKE TYPE 1, FEELS LIKE TYPE 1, BUT ISN'T TYPE 1

Do you have type 1 diabetes? Does a sibling have it? And a parent? An aunt or uncle? A grandparent? Even if you see a strong family line of type 1 diabetes, you may not have it at all—in fact, relatively little of type 1 diabetes is thought to be genetically inherited. Ask your doctor to test your blood for anti-beta-cell antibodies (e.g., GADA, IA-2A, ICA, etc.), a definitive diagnosis for type 1 diabetes. If it's negative, you probably have MODY, or "mature onset diabetes of the youth" (a terrible name).

Unlike typical type 1 diabetes, MODY is a genetic disorder with a fairly clear family inheritance pattern, where genes involved with pro-ducing insulin are mutated and now not working. Importantly, in con-trast to true type 1 diabetes, MODY does not result in the loss of the insulin-producing beta (β) cells of the pancreas—in MODY the β cells are all there; they just don't work right.

Because of the lack of insulin, a patient will indeed manifest with all the same symptoms of type 1 diabetes, such as hyperglycemia, weight loss, polyuria, and feeling faint, thirsty, and hungry. Critically, whereas a person with type 1 diabetes must be treated with insulin, a patient with MODY, depending on the specific gene that's mutated, can be treated with an oral drug and, in some cases, just by changing lifestyle.

So, your family history of type 1 diabetes may not be type 1 diabe-tes after all.

Early physicians didn't have access to modern technology and screening techniques, so it's understandable that they focused on what they could observe. But why keep focusing on glucose into the modern day?

Well, scientifically, glucose is still more easily measured than insulin. To measure glucose, we only need a simple enzyme on a stick, or a basic glucometer, and that technology has existed for roughly 100 years. Insulin, on the other hand, because of its molecular structure and characteristics, is much more difficult to measure. We didn't have a test until the late 1950s, and it required handling radioactive material. (This discovery was so revolutionary that Dr. Rosalyn Yalow received the Nobel Prize for it!) It's simpler today, but still not so easy and not very cheap.

So, even though we can now measure insulin, this advance came about too late—we'd already committed to thinking of diabetes as being a "glucose disease" and, in turn, developed clinical diagnostic values for the disease based entirely on glucose. If you run a quick internet search for "glucose+diabetes," several top results would immediately inform you of the shared clinical values of blood glucose for diabetes types 1 and 2. (Indeed, the values are the same— 126 milligrams per deciliter [mg/dL]—which should seem odd considering the diseases are so different. Excess glucose is the only thing diabetes types 1 and 2 have in common; other than glucose, they are wildly different diseases with very different symptoms and progressions.) Try a similar internet search for insulin, and you'll find plenty of information on insulin *therapy* but almost nothing about the clinical values of *blood* insulin for diabetes. Even as a professional scientist who studies this condition, I have a hard time finding a consensus on insulin values for diabetes.

All of this is interesting, but it still doesn't explain why so many people with insulin resistance are undiagnosed. After all, if we can identify type 2 diabetes by glucose levels, why not insulin resistance (which is also called "prediabetes")? Well, we fail to identify it because *insulin resistance isn't necessarily a hyperglycemic state.* In other words, someone can have insulin resistance and still enjoy perfectly normal blood glucose levels. But which value *won't* be normal in insulin resistance? You guessed it—insulin. If you're insulin resistant, you'll have higher than normal levels of insulin. But of course, the problem is both finding a consensus value for "too much" blood insulin and actually getting your blood insulin measured clinically; it's not part of the standard tests most doctors order.

This is why we can have a scenario where a person is steadily becoming more and more insulin resistant, but the insulin is still working well enough to keep blood glucose in a normal range. This can develop over years, even decades. But because we more typically look at glucose as the problem, we don't recognize there's an issue until the person is so insulin resistant that their insulin, no matter how much they produce, is no longer enough to keep their blood glucose in check. It's at this point, possibly years after the problem started, that we finally notice the disease.

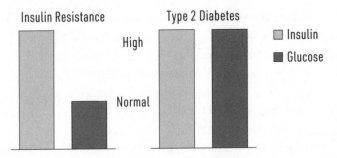

Ultimately, it is unfortunate that history and science played out the way they did. My single greatest frustration is also the reason so many people with insulin resistance are undiagnosed—we look at it wrong. Perhaps if insulin had been the easier-to-measure molecule, we wouldn't have lumped types 1 and 2 diabetes together, and we might have launched a system to identify the disease much earlier—all because we'd have been looking for the more relevant indicator, insulin. After all this, it's no surprise that insulin is a much better predictor of type 2 diabetes than glucose, predicting the problem up to 20 years earlier.[7]

Before moving on, it's helpful to establish a couple points.

First, as mentioned, insulin resistance increases the risk of type 2 diabetes. This is true, but this relationship warrants further clarification. Type 2 diabetes *is* insulin resistance. That is, type 2 diabetes is insulin resistance that has progressed to the point where the body is unable to keep blood glucose levels below the clinically relevant

126 mg/dL. We've known this for almost 100 years; German scientist Wilhelm Falta first proposed the idea in 1931.[8] In other words, any time you hear someone speaking about the evils of diabetes, you can just substitute in "insulin resistance" and it's immediately more accurate. For example, your neighbor doesn't have a family history of diabetes; she has a family history of insulin resistance.

Second, insulin resistance is a hyperinsulinemic state. That means a person with insulin resistance has more insulin in the blood than normal. (This particular point will become highly relevant when we discuss the unfortunate effects of being in this state for prolonged periods.)

As a reminder, note that insulin resistance per se won't kill you; it's just a reliable vehicle that can rapidly get you there by causing other, life-threatening conditions. This means people are experiencing multiple and seemingly diverse health problems that could be improved by addressing one root cause.

Indeed, insulin resistance has a hand in a startling number of very serious chronic diseases, including problems of the head, heart, blood vessels, reproductive organs, and more. Far more than being a mere inconvenience, when left untreated, this is a serious condition. Most people with insulin resistance will ultimately die from heart disease or other cardiovascular complications; others will develop Alzheimer's disease, breast or prostate cancers, or any number of other lethal diseases.

Understanding how insulin resistance causes these disorders is essential to appreciating how important insulin is to our health. That's why we'll spend the next chapters exploring how insulin works throughout the body and just how insulin resistance causes these other conditions. Buckle up—it's a bumpy ride.

CHAPTER 2

Heart Health

HEART DISEASE is *the* leading global cause of death, accounting for more than 30% of disease-related deaths. Naturally, because it is so deadly, there's been much discussion of what causes heart disease. Commonly accused culprits include cigarette smoking, alcohol, dietary cholesterol, lack of exercise, and too much belly fat. But there's not as much focus on insulin resistance. Some circles acknowledge it as a piece of the puzzle, but the truth is more dramatic. It *is* the puzzle—insulin resistance and cardiovascular disorders are almost inseparable. The preeminent physician-scientist Joseph Kraft, who devoted his prolific career to understanding insulin resistance, accurately declared, "Those with cardiovascular disease not identified with diabetes [i.e. insulin resistance] are simply undiagnosed."[1] Where you find one, you find the other.[2] Indeed, the connection is so remarkably strong that there are entire monthly biomedical journals dedicated to the topic.

Now, when we say "heart disease," we don't actually mean one disease in particular; heart disease and cardiovascular disorders are umbrella terms for various conditions that affect our heart and blood vessels. So, "heart disease" might mean elevated blood pressure, thickening of the heart muscle, blood vessel plaques, or another condition. We'll explore several in this chapter.

Hypertension

Having excessively high blood pressure dramatically increases the likelihood of developing heart disease. As the pressure in your blood vessels increases, your heart has to work ever harder to move blood adequately throughout your body and all its tissues. The heart can only meet this strain for so long; if it's not treated, it ultimately results in the heart failing.

There's no debate: insulin resistance and high blood pressure are related. When patients consistently have both, that's evidence of a clear association, and almost all people with hypertension are insulin resistant.[3] This isn't news to medical professionals. However, what *is* news is that they're not just related; we're coming to understand that insulin resistance and high insulin levels directly *cause* high blood pressure.

The reason this is so important is that, as you'll recall, the overwhelming majority of people with insulin resistance don't know they have it. For someone who has just been diagnosed with hypertension, that may be the first evidence they have insulin resistance.

Yet, if you've been diagnosed with high blood pressure, there is a silver lining. Yes, the connection between insulin resistance and hypertension is strong, but that *also* means that as insulin resistance improves, patients generally see quick improvements in their blood pressure.

Over the years, we've come to understand just how insulin resistance, and the accompanying hyperinsulinemia, work in concert to chronically increase blood pressure. Let's take a closer look.[4]

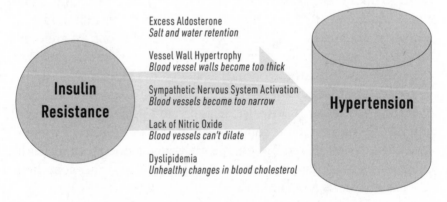

How Insulin Resistance Increases Blood Pressure

Salt and Water Retention

One of the ways that insulin increases blood pressure is through its actions on the hormone aldosterone. Not often discussed, aldosterone has an important role in heart health. Aldosterone is released from the adrenal glands, which are located above the kidneys, and helps to regulate the balance of salt and water in your body. Sodium and chloride, the two parts of salt, are both critical electrolytes that enable all of our body's cells to function properly. Aldosterone signals the kidneys to hold onto sodium and reabsorb it into the blood so it is not expelled through your urine. Thus, if your adrenal glands release more aldosterone into the blood, your body will retain more sodium, and where sodium goes, so, too, does water. This increases the amount of water in the blood, effectively raising the blood volume, and with it, the pressure.

Insulin naturally increases aldosterone levels in the body. So if you have more insulin, as during insulin resistance, its effect on your aldosterone happens abnormally often . . . and, accordingly, it's increasing your blood volume and potentially raising your blood pressure. This very likely explains the remarkably tight association of insulin resistance and hypertension. (It also explains why carbohydrates, which increase insulin more than other nutrients, so effectively increase blood pressure,[5] while dietary fat has no effect[6]—we'll explore dietary factors more in Part II.)

SENSITIVE TO SALT?

Some people develop hypertension due to excess salt intake, but others can eat lots of salt and have no such response. People who develop hypertension from salt consumption are known as "salt-sensitive hypertensives."

In a healthy state, when we eat salt, the body senses the increased salt and "turns aldosterone off" so the kidneys excrete salt and water; this ensures normal blood pressure. However, in the insulin-resistant state, the body has artificially elevated levels of aldosterone. When such a person eats salt, the kidneys disobey normal physiology by retaining salt rather than excreting it along with water. Over time, this leads to an accumulation of body water that increases blood volume and raises blood pressure.[7]

Thicker Blood Vessels

Another way that high insulin leads to high blood pressure is by thickening blood vessel walls.

Blood vessels have several layers, and the innermost layer is lined with cells known as "endothelial cells," or the "endothelium." Remember, insulin is an anabolic hormone—it inherently signals cells to grow bigger, including endothelial cells. This is a healthy and natural response. However, when excess insulin is flowing through the blood, the signal is stronger than normal. As vessel-wall cells grow, the endothelium thickens, and blood vessels begin to narrow.

Imagine a garden hose thickening as water is flowing through it: as the hose walls press in on the flowing water, the pressure inside the hose will climb. This is exactly what happens in the blood vessels as too much insulin excessively stimulates endothelial growth.

Blood Vessels Can't Dilate

Think again about that garden hose with water running through it—if we make the hose larger (not longer), the water will flow more slowly and with less pressure; rather than shooting out, the water will merely be a trickle. Nitric oxide (NO) is a powerful vasodilator, which means it increases the diameter of a blood vessel. Endothelial cells produce NO, which helps the muscle layer that surrounds blood vessels to relax, thereby increasing the size of the vessels. Just like the hose, as vessel diameter increases, the pressure inside plummets. In the body, this pressure-lowering effect is so rapid and potent that we have long used NO, in the form of oral nitroglycerin, to prevent or reverse chest pain by rapidly dilating blood vessels in the heart to increase blood flow. In fact, NO has been shown to be so important in cardiovascular health that scientists exploring its function received the Nobel Prize.

Insulin activates the production of NO in endothelial cells. When insulin flows through a series of blood vessels, it signals those endothelial cells to produce NO, which makes the blood vessels dilate, boosting blood flow to that area.[8] This may be one of the ways that insulin directs the flow and use of nutrients by various tissues. For example, by increasing the blood flow to muscles, insulin helps those muscles receive more nutrients and oxygen.

In contrast to the previous cardiovascular issues we've discussed, where aldosterone and endothelial growth are *overactive* with insulin resistance (because of the hyperinsulinemia), the problem with NO and insulin resistance is that insulin is *less* able to stimulate NO production in endothelial cells. In this scenario, the endothelial cells have become less responsive to insulin's ability to increase NO production. Thus, where insulin once increased blood vessel size and reduced blood pressure, it now has less effect, and blood pressure stays elevated.

Narrow Blood Vessels

Our sympathetic nervous system regulates the body's unconscious actions, including heart rate and heart contraction force, blood vessel size, sweat glands, and more. It is typically referred to as the "fight or flight response" because its events drive the body to action—it "primes the pump" for us to physically perform at our best. Part of this response is to increase blood pressure. We often think of higher blood pressure as a bad thing, but when you're fighting or fleeing for your survival, it is actually very helpful because it can increase the delivery of blood (with all its nutrients and oxygen) to various tissues throughout the body, especially our muscles.

Interestingly, even in the absence of a perceived threat, insulin turns this process on, albeit subtly. However, when you have too much insulin because of resistance, this process is hyperactive—our system is slightly activating the fight-or-flight response to such a degree that we experience an increase in blood pressure that lasts as long as the insulin is elevated.

Unhealthy Changes in Blood Lipids

Lipids are fats or fat-like substances that are present in our blood and tissues. Your body stores fats for future energy use, and when it needs energy, it can break down lipids into fatty acids and burn them like glucose. Dyslipidemia is simply a state of having an abnormal amount of lipids in your blood. Usually, this is defined by simply having *too much* lipid, but it can also indicate that the usual levels of the various lipids are out of order.

The main lipid players are triglycerides (TG), low-density lipoprotein (LDL) cholesterol, and high-density lipoprotein (HDL) cholesterol. Most often, doctors focus on the two cholesterols, and the dogmatic belief is that LDL cholesterol is the villain—many sources refer to HDL as "good" cholesterol and LDL as "bad" cholesterol. While there are certainly data to support that conclusion,[9] many, many studies suggest otherwise[10]; there's little consistent evidence to support the theory that LDL is as lethal as we once believed. This inconsistency may have to do with how we measure it.

Though it's called "low density," LDL cholesterol actually comes in various sizes and densities. Measuring this is getting easier and easier. We've known for decades that our characterization of LDL is more meaningful in predicting heart disease when it is categorized by size and density, which we refer to as a "pattern." There are two patterns, termed A and B, that represent the ends of a spectrum: pattern A refers to an LDL molecule that is larger and less dense, and B refers to the LDL being smaller and denser. Now, for a cholesterol carrier to cause disease, it must pass from the blood and into the blood vessel wall; we can appreciate that a smaller, denser lipoprotein would do this more easily than a bigger one.

If this doesn't make sense, let's use an analogy. Imagine you are standing on a bridge above a river. In your left hand, you're holding a beach ball (LDL A); in your right hand, you're holding a golf ball (LDL B). After you drop both balls into the water, what would happen? The buoyant, less dense beach ball would float along with the river, while (as any golfer knows too well) the denser, less buoyant golf ball would drop to the bottom, bouncing along the riverbed. LDL A and B likely act in a similar way in your blood vessels, with LDL A tending to float along and interact with the blood vessel wall less frequently than LDL B. And, importantly, LDL can only drop off its fats and cholesterol when it bumps into the blood vessel wall. Thus, it's not surprising that people with LDL pattern B are remarkably more likely to experience cardiovascular complications than people with pattern A.[11]

At this point, determining LDL *size* is still not a common part of typical blood tests. If you've had your cholesterol tested recently, you may remember that the lipid panel reported just the main three lipid players: TG, LDL, and HDL. Interestingly, however, we *can* use two of those numbers as a highly accurate indicator of LDL size—a "poor man's" method, if you will. By dividing the level of triglycerides (in mg/dL) by HDL (in mg/dL; TG/HDL), we get a ratio that is surprisingly accurate in predicting LDL size. The lower the ratio (e.g., ~<2.0), the more prevalent the larger, buoyant LDL particles; that is to say, LDL A predominates. But as the ratio climbs (~>2.0), the small, dense LDL B particles are more common.[12] Virtually every blood test will include TG and HDL, which means we can readily get an idea of our individual LDL pattern type without requiring a specialized test.

Low TG:HDL Ratio   High TG:HDL Ratio

HDL

Triglycerides

Pattern A
Reduced development of atherosclerotic plaques

Pattern B
Greater promotion of atherosclerotic plaques

But what does all this have to do with insulin resistance? Insulin selectively drives the production of LDL pattern B from the liver (where almost all cholesterol is made). As insulin levels steadily climb with increasing insulin resistance, the liver is getting the signal to shift the individual toward a pattern B LDL profile.[13] At its simplest, the connection of dyslipidemia to high blood pressure is thought to be due to the accumulation of lipids in the blood vessel walls and the eventual development of an atherosclerotic plaque, reducing vessel diameter. (The actual process is a bit more complicated, as we'll see in the next section.)

STATINS

Statins are one of the most commonly used medications. They are used to reduce cholesterol levels and thus are intended to reduce risk of heart disease. For those with a known genetic defect that increases cholesterol to very high levels (e.g., familial hypercholesterolemia), this might indeed be the case.[14] However, for people without this disease and who have never had a heart attack, yet are at high risk based on conventional blood lipid markers, such as LDL levels, statins provide remarkably little benefit,[15] possibly because statins actually appear to increase the ratio of pattern B to pattern A LDL cholesterol.[16]

Independent of its effect on cholesterol, statins have side effects relevant to insulin resistance: postmenopausal women who take statins may increase their risk of developing type 2 diabetes by up to 50%.[17] We are gaining an ever-clearer picture of how statins cause insulin resistance. While some of the effect may be statins damaging muscle tissue,[18] statins also block the cell's responsiveness to insulin and promote the release of hormones that increase glucose in the blood (making insulin work harder to lower glucose).[19]

Atherosclerosis

Atherosclerosis is the most essential process in the development of heart disease.[20] Our great fear of cholesterol stems from the theory that it leads to atherosclerosis, a process wherein the blood vessels become hardened and narrowed (as just mentioned).[21] But let's look at this process more closely.

As described in the last section, to be pathogenic, cholesterol must pass into the blood vessel wall. However, cholesterol being deposited in the endothelium isn't *in itself* the cause of disease. When they enter the endothelium, cholesterol and fats are benign—they appear to elicit no negative response. Indeed, the cells that line blood vessels, like all other cells in the body, *need* cholesterol and fats to maintain healthy function! Nevertheless, the lipids may not be benign for long. In certain people, something happens to the cholesterol and fats to make them noxious.

The switch is flipped when the fats and/or cholesterol are oxidized, which happens when oxidative stress is high. Once that happens, white blood cells called macrophages engulf the oxidized lipid to prevent it from oxidizing other parts of cells. (The name *macrophage* comes from the Greek for "big eater," which is apt considering how these cells work: they swallow up and digest pathogens, foreign substances, and cellular debris.) Over time, the macrophage will become loaded with oxidized fat or cholesterol; the lipid-laden cell is known as a "foam cell" due to its foamy appearance under a microscope. This foam cell then recruits help by releasing proteins to signal more macrophages to come to the area (known as an inflammatory response). The newcomers also become foam cells over time, worsening the problem. Eventually, this mix of foam cells and lipids becomes the core of the atherosclerotic plaque.

At the risk of complicating the problem, as much as the focus has been on cholesterol, it's more valid (and fair) to spread the blame to include noncholesterol fats. In particular, the polyunsaturated fat called linoleic acid (very common in seed oils, such as soybean oil) is the most readily oxidized fat—far more so than cholesterol—and is likely a main culprit.[22] In fact, when cholesterol gets oxidized, it's often due to a linoleic acid being bound to a cholesterol molecule[23]— as though our neutral cholesterol is forced to give the naughty child, oxidized linoleic acid, a piggyback ride. Nevertheless, even here, insulin resistance is relevant.

Insulin resistance is an important risk factor for atherosclerosis.[24] This is likely because insulin resistance stimulates the two main variables thought to be involved in this disease. We already discussed one: the role of insulin in increasing LDL pattern B subtype; LDL B can carry the problem fats, like linoleic acid. The other variable is oxidative stress. Insulin resistance seems to increase oxidative stress[25]; later, we'll see that it goes both ways, and that oxidative stress also increases insulin resistance.

Inflammation

Various markers of inflammation, especially the increasingly well-known C-reactive protein, more accurately predict cardiovascular disorders than cholesterol levels.[26] Remarkably, whereas insulin elicits anti-inflammatory actions in an insulin-sensitive person (with normal levels of insulin),[27] insulin activates inflammation in insulin-resistant people (with high levels of insulin).[28]

This matters. A lot. Implicating insulin resistance as a cause of inflammation places insulin resistance at ground zero for heart disease—it's waging war on the blood vessels by doing everything to promote atherosclerosis. First, insulin resistance increases blood pressure, increasing the likelihood of blood vessel damage. Next, it increases lipid deposition in blood vessel walls. Finally, insulin resistance increases inflammation, promoting the ongoing infiltration of the blood vessel with macrophages, which become increasingly laden with oxidized lipids, changing into foam cells. Altogether, these events, each spurred on separately by insulin resistance, culminate to form an atherosclerotic plaque. With all this in mind, it's little surprise that insulin can *directly* promote foam-cell formation in blood vessels![29]

Cardiomyopathy

A separate class of cardiovascular disorders specifically involves the heart muscle, or myocardium. With cardiomyopathy, the muscles of the heart become unable to generate enough force to pump blood throughout the body's countless vessels. There are several types of cardiomyopathy, but they are all generally classified by the structural changes in the heart, including:

- dilated cardiomyopathy, where the heart is "ballooned out";
- hypertrophic cardiomyopathy, where the heart muscle is too thick and prevents adequate filling; and
- restrictive cardiomyopathy, where the heart muscle becomes scarred and stiff.

Collectively, these cardiomyopathies are sometimes referred to as "nonischemic heart failure," meaning that it's not a lack of blood flow (e.g., atherosclerosis or a heart attack) causing the heart to fail.

Of the three main types, insulin resistance has been most strongly associated with dilated cardiomyopathy, or DCM.[30] Heart muscle cells rely on glucose for their main fuel. With DCM, the heart muscle (or myocardium) becomes dilated, meaning it stretches and gets thinner. As this continues, the heart muscle doesn't contract normally and can't pump blood very well; the theory is that over the course of the disorder, the myocardium becomes ever more reliant on glucose to keep working. However, insulin resistance compromises the heart's ability to take in and use glucose; because of this metabolic change, the heart begins to suffer from a relative lack of energy and nutrients.[31]

Although there's not as much evidence as there is for insulin resistance and DCM, some studies indicate insulin resistance may play a role in the development of hypertrophic cardiomyopathy.[32] (That's not especially surprising—nothing is at this point, right?) Very likely, the chronically elevated insulin drives the growth of the myocardium, making it too thick to allow the heart chambers to fill with blood.

By now, I hope it is clear: though we often blame other factors, there is no single variable more relevant to heart disease than insulin resistance. Any successful efforts to reduce our high risk of heart disease *must* address it. When we acknowledge the central role of insulin resistance, we start resolving the fundamental causes, rather than symptoms (which is all medications can do). As much as worldwide efforts to stem heart disease have tried, the longer we overlook insulin resistance, the worse the problem will get.

CHAPTER 3

The Brain and Neurological Disorders

J UST 20 YEARS AGO, medical texts listed the brain as an organ that had no response to insulin. How times have changed! Since then, we've had an explosion of research in this area. We now know that insulin regulates *many* processes in the brain—and we're discovering more and more that show how insulin resistance threatens brain health.

Like every cell in the body, brain cells have insulin receptors— they sense and respond to insulin, which helps them function. Insulin stimulates the brain to take up glucose for fuel[1] and helps our brain cells grow and survive.[2] The hormone also plays a role in regulating our appetite and how we use energy; when the brain senses increased insulin in the body (which occurs after a meal), our appetite will wane. Due to its additional actions in the brain, insulin also alters reproductive hormones (which we will explore later).[3]

What's more, insulin plays an important role in learning and memory formation.[4] One remarkable study in rats looked at an experimental model of type 1 diabetes, wherein some of the rats couldn't make insulin. The rats with type 1 diabetes failed to learn a maze as well as the rats in the control group with typical insulin production. However, upon receiving insulin, the learning and memory of the animals with diabetes improved.[5]

All of this simply suggests the importance of insulin in normal brain function. Problems arise when you have too much insulin or when the brain fails to respond to insulin[6]—in other words, when the brain becomes insulin resistant.[7] When we talk about insulin resistance, it's tempting to only think of a few tissues becoming insulin resistant, like the muscles or the liver. However, researchers appreciate more and more that the brain becomes insulin resistant concurrently with the rest of the tissues. Moreover, actual brain structure requires healthy insulin sensitivity; prolonged insulin resistance physically alters the brain. A recent study found that for every 10 years of insulin resistance, the brain looks two years older than the brain of an insulin-sensitive person of the same age.[8] As an obvious consequence, normal brain function becomes impaired. Less responsiveness to insulin may lead us to overeat, contributing to weight gain; it also compromises our short-term learning and may damage our long-term memory.[9] This link between insulin and the brain has important implications for our health and ability to live independently.

Not only that, insulin resistance can inflict profound harm on brain physiology, increasing the risk of developing severe brain-related diseases. In this chapter, we'll take a look at the link between insulin and diseases of the brain and central nervous system, beginning with the most common, Alzheimer's disease.

A New Understanding of Alzheimer's

As much as we've seen just how relevant insulin resistance is in prominent brain diseases, we still have much to learn about dementia. The term "dementia" refers to a loss of memory and intellectual function that compromises daily life; various disorders qualify as dementia, and Alzheimer's is the most common.

We don't yet fully understand the causes and nature of Alzheimer's disease, and our corresponding inability to prevent or cure it has resulted in its rapidly becoming the most common neurological disorder, accounting for up to 80% of all dementia cases and affecting roughly 30 million people worldwide.[10] If current trends continue, this number is expected to double every 20 years.[11] Despite its prevalence, we still have little understanding of how to diagnose and treat—not to mention prevent—the disease. In fact, our understanding is so vague that we can only diagnose it with certainty by dissecting the brain post mortem. What's becoming increasingly clear, however, is the remarkable contribution of insulin resistance to the disease—it's so relevant that it has given rise to a new term for Alzheimer's: "type 3 diabetes."[12]

Interestingly, physicians and scientists have been aware of the Alzheimer's–insulin resistance connection for decades, though these early observations were thought to be because Alzheimer's patients had a relatively sedentary lifestyle. In other words, biomedical professionals thought people with Alzheimer's were developing insulin resistance because they couldn't get out and exercise. However, additional inquiry revealed that early-stage Alzheimer's patients had similar levels of physical activity and lifestyles to healthy non-Alzheimer's patients, but still were more insulin resistant. With mounting evidence, the connection became harder to ignore.

Alzheimer's disease is a complicated disorder that undoubtedly involves mechanisms we're not yet aware of. However, in early stages of Alzheimer's research, a general consensus formed around the idea that two main features of the disease are accumulations of plaques and tangles in the brain.

In Alzheimer's, the theory goes, the brain accumulates plaques made up of amyloid beta peptide (Aβ). Amyloids are protein bits that the body produces normally. When they build up into clusters called plaques, they may disrupt normal brain function, including memory, mood, motor function, and learning.

Because these Aβ plaques are so harmful, our brains have built-in processes that help prevent them from forming. The most prominent preventive mechanism is apolipoprotein E (APOE), a lipoprotein that has many functions in the body. In the brain, it carries essential cholesterol to our neurons and furthers the breakdown of Aβ plaques—when it's working right. There are three types of genes for APOE, however, and roughly 15% of all people have a version known as APOE4, which fails to perform this antiplaque duty at typical levels. People with APOE4 are roughly 10 to 30 times more likely to develop Alzheimer's disease by their mid-70s.[13] Because of this, when studies have explored risk factors for getting Alzheimer's disease, having APOE4 is usually the most significant variable. For example, a research group in Finland performed a survey of risk factors for Alzheimer's disease across a broad population.[14] Unsurprisingly, having the APOE4 phenotype was the most highly significant variable in people with Alzheimer disease (p = 0.0001, for those readers who care about the statistical strength!). Other significant variables included age (p = .005) and education level (p = .002; a secondary benefit of attending school, although this may largely be a function of simply keeping one's mind active and frequently challenged).[15] After that? The next most statistically significant variable wasn't hypertension (p = .31), history of stroke (p = .59), or smoking status (p = .47). It was fasting insulin (p = .0005). That's right—your fasting insulin carries a stronger statistical significance than your age! Remarkably, every single marker of insulin resistance in this study was statistically significant with Alzheimer's disease, including various blood glucose and insulin measurements.

Insulin may contribute directly to Aβ plaque accumulation. In one study, researchers infused healthy older adults with insulin. They found that this artificial, acute state of high insulin increased Aβ in the participants' cerebrospinal fluid, even more dramatically so in elderly patients.[16] But producing Aβ alone may not be sufficient to affect Alzheimer's disease risk; location matters. With Alzheimer's disease, Aβ plaques accumulate in the spaces between nerves in the brain, not in the nerves themselves. And sure enough, insulin increases Aβ *release* from brain nerves,[17] increasing its accumulation outside and between brain cells.

Neurofibrillary tangles are thought to be another key feature of Alzheimer's disease. Tau is a protein that acts to maintain normal nerve structure. With Alzheimer's disease, tau becomes overactive and, like a rambunctious child, somewhat frenetic. This means tau doesn't do its job as well; instead of maintaining nerve structure, tau now twists the nerves, creating neurofibrillary tangles.

Even here, insulin is relevant. Normal insulin signaling in the brain inhibits the activity of tau.[18] So, when this signaling is compromised (as it is with insulin resistance), tau becomes overactive, potentially leading to neurofibrillary tangles.[19]

In the face of such evidence supporting the role for Aβ plaques and neurofibrillary tangles, it's hard to believe there might be an alternative theory to explain the disease's origins. But a recent study found plaques and tangles in the brains of elderly people who had *no* signs of dementia[20]—clearly, something else is going on, requiring another perspective.

The alternative theory is out there, and it's focused on alterations in the brain's metabolic workings. (As you may have guessed by now, insulin *still* plays a role.)

The brain has tremendous energy demands. At rest, it's one of the most metabolically active tissues in our body (several times more than muscle), and so is very sensitive to any energy deprivation. It's a high-performance engine that starts to sputter as fuel gets low. The brain of a person in a "fed state"—having eaten a conventional meal—receives 100% of its energy from glucose, as opposed to less than half during a fasted state (with the rest coming from something called "ketones," which we'll discuss later).[21] In a typical Western diet, the frequency with which we eat (every few hours) and the types of foods we choose (often highly processed) create a constant fed state. This complete glucose reliance creates a frightening problem. The brain's inability to get enough glucose is a cardinal feature of Alzheimer's disease. As in our muscles, insulin facilitates the movement of glucose into the brain. However, as the brain becomes progressively insulin resistant, it becomes less and less able to obtain enough glucose to meet its energy demands.[22] So, like an engine running on empty, the brain doesn't work as well. This phenomenon is known as "glucose hypometabolism," and the greater the degree a person has it, the more rapid the onset of clinical Alzheimer's disease. The decline generally goes: less brain insulin sensitivity → less brain glucose uptake → less brain energy → compromised brain function.

Because of its increasing prominence, we are focusing on and learning more about Alzheimer's than ever before. While some older theories, like plaques and tangles, are losing ground, our discoveries into the metabolic origins of Alzheimer's, including insulin's key role, are presenting new and better approaches to detection and treatment. Yet remarkably, insulin resistance doesn't stop there; in addition to its part in Alzheimer's, insulin resistance is also involved in other forms of dementia.

Vascular Dementia

After Alzheimer's disease, the vascular form of dementia is the second most common. Its symptoms are very similar to Alzheimer's; however, vascular dementia occurs because the brain suffers from insufficient blood flow. But the two disorders are related—accumulated plaques in the brain may hurt blood vessels, too. If the plaques-and-tangles theory is correct, Alzheimer's disease may contribute to vascular dementia.[23]

Recall the cardiovascular disorders that we covered earlier. We've already seen that insulin resistance extensively influences blood vessel function, so you might expect a strong association between insulin resistance and vascular dementia. Sure enough, the Honolulu-Asia Aging Program, which followed almost 10,000 adult men for more than 20 years, observed that subjects with insulin resistance have about twice the risk of developing vascular dementia compared with insulin-sensitive subjects.[24] This is very likely because of a combination of factors we discussed in relation to high blood pressure (such as altered nitric oxide production, thickening blood vessel walls, and other mechanisms we discussed in chapter two). Whatever the mechanism, the evidence is compelling: the cardiovascular complications that arise from insulin resistance don't just create heart problems, they might also lead to vascular dementia.

Parkinson's Disease

Parkinson's disease is a brain disorder that is most evident in altering patients' ability to control their bodily movements. On top of motor symptoms like slow movement, stiff limbs, and tremors, it can also lead to other issues like depression, sleep disorders, fatigue, and cognitive changes. Although around 60,000 people are diagnosed annually with Parkinson's, we only poorly understand its causes, and we have no way to prevent or cure it.

Most people with Parkinson's develop dementia as their disease progresses. A main feature of this dementia is the accrual of proteins called "Lewy bodies" in the brain. However, even more critical is the loss of dopamine-producing neurons. Parkinson's disease develops in a part of the brain called the substantia nigra, a structure in the midbrain that controls motor movement and reward functions. The cells here produce dopamine, and when they begin to die, the loss of dopamine causes movement issues.

Insulin is known to alter dopamine in the brain,[25] which provides a direct and causal relationship between insulin and Parkinson's. Furthermore, one study found that by lowering insulin in rats, dopamine receptors in their brains increased by 35%,[26] and a study in humans found that the most insulin-resistant people had the lowest rates of dopamine production in their brains.[27]

While the consensus with Parkinson disease and insulin resistance is that the insulin problem drives the dopamine problem, there is evidence of the reverse.[28] In other words, usually changes in insulin lead to changes in dopamine receptors, but some studies have found that altering dopamine leads to changes in insulin.

In rodent and human experiments, improving dopamine signaling elicits an improvement in metabolic function, while dampening the signaling makes metabolic function worse—and can even create insulin resistance. The evidence in humans is fascinating. People who were treated with antipsychotic medications, which block dopamine receptors, develop insulin resistance and gain weight. In fact, up to 40% of people treated with antipsychotics may develop type 2 diabetes within five years.[29] Once people stop taking the medication, the insulin resistance disappears within weeks.[30]

Regardless of the factors directly linking insulin with Parkinson's disease, a clear association exists. Up to 30% of patients with Parkinson's disease have type 2 diabetes, with possibly up to 80% having insulin resistance (or prediabetes).[31]

HUNTINGTON'S DISEASE

There is very little substantive evidence suggesting a causal relationship between insulin resistance and Huntington's disease. Nonetheless, I consider the disease worth mentioning, because people with Huntington's disease are much more likely to be insulin resistant than non-Huntington's patients, despite having similar characteristics (age, body composition, etc.).[32] In fact, in a well-controlled study, people with Huntington's disease were almost 10 times more likely to have symptoms of insulin resistance compared with healthy people.[33]

Huntington's disease is a very clear genetic disease, based on a person inheriting the huntingtin gene, which over time leads to devastating damage to muscle and mind. Studies of Huntington's disease involve particular rodents that develop the disease by having their DNA tweaked to include the human huntingtin gene. Interestingly, these mice, along with developing Huntington's disease, become insulin resistant within weeks.[34]

Migraine Headaches

Among the most common neurological disorders, migraine headaches affect roughly 18% of US adults. A study of middle-aged women found that those who had insulin resistance were twice as likely to have regular migraines.[35] A separate study in men and women found that insulin levels were significantly higher in people who experience migraines compared with people who don't.[36] Looking at this another way, when treated with an insulin-sensitizing medication, over half of a group of 32 people with regular migraines experienced a significant reduction in migraine frequency.[37]

Like Alzheimer's disease, part of the problem with migraines could be a "running on empty" scenario where the brain isn't getting enough fuel[38]; when insulin isn't working, glucose can't get to the brain.

Neuropathy

Now that we've established the relevance of insulin resistance in healthy brain function, it's important to remember that the brain is sort of a bundle of nerves, and these nerves communicate with nerves spread throughout the body. Just like the nerves in the brain, those outside the brain are affected by insulin resistance. The nerve damage that accompanies diabetes—the burning, tingling sensation in the limbs, particularly the feet—is so commonly associated with type 2 diabetes that it's considered a staple of the disease. This diabetes-induced neuropathy has long been seen as a consequence of the hyperglycemia that clinically identifies type 2 diabetes. However, recent findings are challenging this notion; while hyperglycemia is undoubtedly relevant to neuropathy, the problem appears to start before blood glucose changes, suggesting something other than glucose is to blame. Of course, that "something" is insulin resistance. Nerves, like every other cell in the body, respond to insulin, which determines how the nerve takes in and uses energy. As the nerve becomes insulin resistant, its ability to maintain normal function is compromised, eventually causing neuropathy.[39]

We now know that insulin is relevant to most brain-related chronic diseases. Because the brain needs a lot of energy to function, it needs a reliable fuel. When the brain becomes insulin resistant, access to this fuel becomes limited. And that's relevant even before disease sets in. We've only just begun to understand all the roles insulin plays in the brain and central nervous system. It influences appetite, helps with memory, regulates dopamine, and more. Bottom line: A healthy brain requires healthy insulin sensitivity.

Brain and other nervous disorders are sobering health concerns; losing control of your body is a terrifying scenario. However, by acknowledging the role that insulin resistance plays in these conditions, we introduce a new perspective not only on identifying the disorders but possibly for slowing their progress or even preventing them.

CHAPTER 4

Reproductive Health

BECAUSE YOU'RE NOT MY TEENAGE CHILD, you'll allow me to freely discuss sex and its wondrous intricacies. Of course, to keep our species alive, humans, like all other organisms, reproduce. Some of us do this quite well (just ask my parents—I have 12 siblings . . .), while others may suffer the heartache that usually accompanies infertility. Regardless of the situation, among the essential components of reproductive health are the sex hormones produced by the primary sex glands (testes in men, ovaries in women), with some involvement from the brain. The brain and sex glands, known as gonads, interact to properly orchestrate the many events in men and women that must happen to allow reproduction. However, you might be surprised to learn that a humble hormone from the pancreas plays an important role as well.

The connection between insulin resistance and reproductive disorders may be the most unexpected one that we cover. Most people would never imagine that insulin plays *any* role in reproduction, let alone an essential one. And yet, insulin is absolutely necessary for normal reproduction—which may be evidence of a simple yet profound link between our metabolic and reproductive function. After all, reproducing is risky business! It wouldn't be prudent to bring offspring into a dangerous or unhealthy situation, such as a period of starvation. Insulin, then, acts as a signal that tells our brain if our environment is metabolically safe. Normal insulin levels suggest the potential parent-to-be is healthy and their diet is sufficient to grow a fetus and even raise a newborn.

The fact that we need insulin for healthy reproduction is clear. Experiments with rodents have revealed that a lack of insulin leads to changes in brain and gonad function that decrease reproductive processes.[1] But too much insulin isn't any better than too little. (Remember, insulin resistance is almost always a state of hyperinsulinemia—the pancreas is producing more insulin than normal in an effort to increase insulin's actions.) Insulin-resistant men[2] and women[3] are more likely to be infertile than their insulin-sensitive counterparts. Additionally, insulin-resistant children are more likely to experience alterations in puberty.[4]

Exactly why this happens is fascinating and illustrates both how delicately fertility is regulated and the ways metabolic processes drive reproductive processes. In this chapter, we'll take a look at the many sexual and reproductive complications that can arise when men, women, and kids have insulin troubles.

Insulin and Women's Reproductive Health

Reproduction is a complex process in women. Throughout a woman's menstrual cycle, a series of hormonal changes lead to the development and eventual release of an egg, a process called ovulation, which generally happens each month. If she becomes pregnant, a woman's reproductive capacities also include developing and sustaining the growing baby. And even after birth, her job isn't done—her body continues to change, including the production of breast milk and other shifts that affect reproduction.

For women, reproduction involves a great deal of change and growth and demands a lot of energy. Perhaps for these reasons, women's fertility and reproductive health appear to be much more intimately linked with insulin and insulin resistance than men's.

Before we talk about the pathological side of insulin and reproductive disorders in women, I have to highlight the interesting—and normal—relationship between insulin and pregnancy. Insulin is a growth signal, turning on anabolic processes to increase the size of our cells and sometimes even their number. The pregnant body needs to grow, and insulin helps that happen. Insulin helps the placenta grow,[5] helps breast tissue develop in preparation for lactation,[6] and even helps ensure Mom has enough energy available for the demanding process of pregnancy by increasing her body's inclination to store fat. In fact, to facilitate this, insulin receptors are increased in a woman's fat tissue at the onset of pregnancy, then return to normal levels after birth.[7] Maternal fat tissue will grow more readily during pregnancy because of fat tissue's heightened responsiveness to insulin than at other times in life.

Pregnancy is one of very few instances where insulin resistance appears to be a *normal* and even helpful event. Yes, pregnancy is a naturally insulin-resistant state. The average, healthy woman will become roughly half as insulin sensitive at the end of her pregnancy as she was at the beginning.[8] And in this case, insulin resistance is a good thing! The technical term for this is "physiological insulin resistance"—meaning it's insulin resistance with a purpose. As a pregnant woman's body becomes insulin resistant, insulin levels increase (although it's just as likely that her body becomes insulin resistant because of the elevated insulin levels, described later), which drives tissue growth, such as the placenta.

But the elevated insulin levels in pregnancy do more than prepare the mother-to-be; even more important, insulin also helps stimulate growth and development of the growing baby.[9] So, just as the elevated insulin is preparing the maternal body for optimal pregnancy function, it is also giving the fetus a critical growth signal.

That said, while insulin resistance is a natural occurrence in pregnancy, it can have other implications for women's reproductive health, including fertility issues, polycystic ovarian syndrome, gestational diabetes, preeclampsia, and more.

Gestational Diabetes

The most obvious reproduction-related disorder with insulin resistance in women is gestational diabetes mellitus. This happens when the woman becomes sufficiently insulin resistant during the course of her pregnancy that her insulin is not enough to keep blood glucose at normal levels. At this point, the normal, physiological insulin resistance has become pathological; the fine line between these two states is glucose control.

Gestational diabetes can happen to any pregnant woman, though the usual risk factors that apply to insulin resistance are the most relevant. We'll get into risk factors in more detail in Part II, but for gestational diabetes, they include pre-pregnancy body weight, age, family history of diabetes, and ethnicity (with those of Asian, Hispanic, and Middle Eastern descent having the highest risk; they're all ethnicities with greater risk of insulin resistance).[10]

Unfortunately, even if the woman had no evidence of insulin resistance or type 2 diabetes before pregnancy, developing gestational diabetes increases her likelihood of developing type 2 diabetes later in life. In fact, on average, her risk of developing type 2 diabetes is sevenfold higher when compared with a woman who did not have gestational diabetes during pregnancy.[11]

Preeclampsia

More severe insulin resistance during pregnancy, which usually manifests as gestational diabetes, increases the risk of developing one of the most lethal pregnancy disorders, preeclampsia—a dangerous change in kidney function. Women who develop more dramatic insulin resistance during early pregnancy are significantly more likely to develop preeclampsia during the second half.[12]

The connection between the two disorders is not fully understood, but it very likely has to do with at least some of the blood pressure problems that arise from insulin resistance, including activation of the sympathetic nervous system and reduced nitric oxide production[13] (for a refresher, refer to chapter two).

However it may happen, the altered blood pressure with insulin resistance creates a situation where blood flow to tissues in the mother, including the placenta, is less than ideal.[14] When it's not getting enough blood, the placenta creates a signal protein called vascular endothelial growth factor (VEGF) for itself and the rest of the body. VEGF stimulates the formation of blood vessels, and in releasing this protein, the placenta is trying to increase the amount of blood that it receives.[15] In a healthy pregnancy, this is exactly what happens; the placenta needs more blood and VEGF helps it happen. But in the case of preeclampsia, the placenta inexplicably releases a second protein called the soluble VEGF receptor, which sticks to VEGF and prevents it from working. So, even though the placenta is making VEGF, the protein can't do anything.

Not only does this scenario hurt the placenta (by not letting it create new blood vessels), but the kidneys suffer a serious setback—they need the VEGF that the placenta makes. The kidneys normally use VEGF to maintain normal blood filtration, which is their main job and absolutely necessary for health. When the kidneys don't get enough VEGF, they start to lose their functionality. They stop filtering properly, and toxins and excess water start to accumulate in the blood. Higher blood volume via excess water is the main cause of increased blood pressure (as we saw in chapter two). But the toxins are the more dangerous feature, potentially leading to seizures and death as they affect the brain. Meanwhile, the kidneys' lack of VEGF also causes them to become "leaky," allowing protein from the blood to spill into the urine. This is why we monitor not only the blood pressure of women with preeclampsia, but also the amount of urinary protein as an indicator of kidney health.

If it isn't caught early and treated, preeclampsia can lead to liver or kidney failure and future heart issues for the mother. For the baby, less blood flow to the placenta means the fetus gets less food and oxygen—leading to lower-than-normal birthweight. The only real solution for preeclampsia is to remove the placenta, which means removing the baby as soon as it is developed enough to deliver safely. That means inducing labor or a very early caesarean section to protect the mother's health.

Over- and Underweight Babies

Being born on either end of the weight spectrum can have consequences later in life, and having a mother with hyperinsulinemia and insulin resistance has a surprisingly strong influence on this.

Before we go on, I want to clarify that when I refer to a newborn's weight in this section, I don't mean a baby that is naturally smaller or bigger because of family genetics. I'm discussing the situation when, all things considered, a baby is born smaller or larger than anticipated.

A mother's metabolic health and the health of her baby are closely connected. Some of the strongest evidence for this comes from the Dutch Famine Study, which tracked the health of people who were conceived during the Dutch famine of 1944–1945 at the end of World War II.[16] The researchers were able to explore the effects the famine had on these individuals depending on whether it had occurred early, late, or in the middle of the mother's pregnancy. Individuals whose mothers endured famine at the beginning of pregnancy were significantly more likely to be obese later in life compared with normal. Importantly, these observations weren't necessarily associated with the infant being born larger or smaller than normal—it was independent of newborn body weight. (As we will see in later chapters, obesity and insulin resistance are closely connected.)

For a mother with more dramatic pregnancy insulin resistance (such as maternal gestational diabetes and/or polycystic ovarian syndrome—more on that later), the most common result is that the infant is born with a higher birthweight than normal. The fetus has developed in an insulin- and possibly glucose-rich environment, thriving beyond what is typical. This may seem benign, but it has lasting effects. These infants are roughly 40% more likely to be obese and have metabolic complications in their teenage years and beyond.[17]

On the other end of the spectrum are infants born below the normal and expected birthweight (common when the mother develops preeclampsia[18]). It might be tempting to assume that any child born with a high birthweight is much more likely to become obese and insulin resistant than a normal-birthweight baby and certainly more than a low-birthweight (LBW) baby. But it's not so simple.

While individuals with a high birthweight do indeed have an increased likelihood of obesity and insulin resistance later in childhood,[19] the risk is actually greater in those with LBW. Paradoxically, just like the high-birthweight infants, these children are more likely than average to develop obesity and metabolic disorders later in life. The metabolic complications of LBW have been particularly well documented in the UK, where researchers have consistently observed that children born thin don't stay that way for long.[20] Yes, it's true—infants born below the normal weight are the most likely to become obese and insulin resistant.[21] This trend can start to appear as early as four years old—by this age, the child has often caught up to normal-weight peers and begins to surpass them in weight, though it can happen later in the teenage years as well and last into late adulthood.[22] A part of this effect may be related to the physical stress of being born LBW and potentially confounding events surrounding the birth[23] (we'll discuss how stress connects to insulin resistance on pages 98–99).

WHAT ABOUT DAD?

The overwhelming majority of research on neonatal metabolic complications has focused on the role of the mother's insulin and metabolic health. The relatively smaller focus on the *father's* insulin and metabolic health has yielded conflicting results.[24] However, studies that track and explore insulin resistance and other metabolic parameters of the offspring, not just birthweight, support the idea that paternal insulin resistance matters; if Dad has insulin resistance, it's one more trait baby may inherit.[25]

Low Breast Milk Supply

Independent of any effect on baby's development and mother's health, maternal insulin resistance can also affect the mother's ability to nurse. A 2000 study of mothers with gestational diabetes revealed that women with the worst insulin resistance were likely to have the lowest milk supply.[26]

Interestingly, if a new mother has a problem breastfeeding, she also has a stumbling block to the built-in solution for improving her insulin resistance. Breastfeeding is an effective method of increasing the mother's postnatal insulin sensitivity.[27] So, having insulin resistance could make it more difficult to take advantage of a natural way to reverse the insulin resistance of pregnancy.

Polycystic Ovarian Syndrome

Polycystic ovarian syndrome (PCOS) is the most common cause of female infertility, affecting approximately 10 million women worldwide. As the name suggests, the ovaries of the affected woman become burdened with cysts, resulting in highly painful ovaries that grow to several times their normal size. At its very core, PCOS is a disease of too much insulin, an inseparable and causal factor.

As I mentioned earlier, female fertility is an elaborate orchestra of hormones. In the first part of a woman's menstrual cycle, her estrogen levels are low. A small but important part of the brain called the hypothalamus sends a signal to the pituitary gland, also located in the brain, which then releases follicle-stimulating hormone (FSH). FSH tells a few of the follicles in the ovaries to develop into mature eggs. One of the eggs becomes dominant. As the follicles mature, they send a massive increase in estrogens from the ovaries, which tells the hypothalamus and pituitary that there's an egg ready for release. The pituitary gland then releases luteinizing hormone (LH). This surge in LH causes the dominant, mature egg to emerge through the ovary—this is ovulation. With ovulation, a hormonal signal goes to the remaining developing eggs and causes their degradation, and they subsequently disappear from the ovaries.

Did you get all that? As I said, this process is complex! Ultimately, what's important to know is that the process of allowing one egg to become dominant and eventually be ovulated is governed by specific hormone fluctuations. If these waves of hormones are disrupted, it creates a problem.

So how exactly is insulin involved? Well, ovaries, like every tissue, respond to insulin. Perhaps one of the more unexpected ways they do so is by inhibiting estrogen production. All estrogens were once androgens; during production, an enzyme called aromatase converts androgens ("male hormones"), such as testosterone, into estrogens ("female hormones"). (This process occurs in both men and women, by the way.) But too much insulin inhibits aromatase. As the enzyme's actions are dialed down, androgens fail to convert to estrogens at the necessary levels, estrogen production becomes lower than normal, and androgens become higher than normal.

Estrogens have countless effects throughout the body; one of the main ones in women is their role in the menstrual cycle. As we just saw, production of estrogens increases dramatically around midway through the cycle. This spike in estrogens signals the brain, which increases the level of LH production, resulting in ovulation and the eventual degradation of the other developing eggs. If this mid-cycle estrogen bump doesn't happen owing to insulin resistance, ovulation doesn't happen, and the ovaries retain and accumulate the eggs.

Beyond its effects on estrogens, insulin may also directly act on the brain to block normal LH production. LH production usually comes in pulses—periods of increased then decreased production. Insulin appears to prevent this pattern, which may disrupt normal fertility.

Insulin's effects on sex hormones go beyond fertility issues. With PCOS, relatively fewer androgens are being converted to estrogen, resulting in high androgen levels. Higher androgens can lead to more and coarser facial and body hair and male-pattern baldness in women. Last, high insulin alone, independent of sex hormones, often increases the presence of dark skin patches called acanthosis nigricans (described further in chapter six), a common feature of PCOS.

Problems with Fertility Treatments

As you might have guessed, considering the various reproductive disorders insulin resistance causes, many resistant women end up seeking fertility treatments. Unfortunately, even here, insulin resistance insists its presence be noted.

Before we talk about treatments, I want to acknowledge that insulin sensitivity has a direct positive effect on women's fertility. Reducing insulin levels and improving insulin sensitivity, whether by weight loss or use of insulin-sensitizing drugs, increases natural ovulation in the absence of any fertility-drug intervention.[28]

One of the most common therapies to improve female fertility is treatment with clomiphene, which alters estrogens to induce ovulation. However, insulin-resistant women with PCOS respond poorly to the drug and typically require higher doses, which can lead to negative side effects.[29] In fact, measuring blood insulin in the woman with PCOS is the most reliable indicator for predicting her responsiveness to clomiphene—the lower the insulin, the higher her response.

If female fertility is a complicated orchestra of hormones, insulin is the conductor. Abnormal crescendos and decrescendos of fertility hormones throughout the menstrual cycle, including estrogens, FSH, and LH, are just following the conductor. If a woman is able to get her insulin under control, often the fertility hormones will follow, and the most common forms of infertility, as just outlined, are, like a bad song, simply turned off.

Insulin and Men's Reproductive Health

In contrast to the complexities of female fertility, reproductive health in men is a (relatively) straightforward matter. The primary problem with male infertility is low sperm counts or poor sperm quality.

Secondary problems, far less frequent, often include anatomical problems or genetic defects. In this section, we'll focus on two big problems that can arise with insulin resistance: sperm production and
erectile dysfunction. Because insulin resistance is related to both of
these problems, let's first look at its association with testosterone.

We have a cultural obsession with testosterone. It is now common
to hear men talk about being diagnosed with "low T" and blame it for
their other health complications, including lack of energy and inability
to lose weight. Many are inclined to think that the low testosterone is
the cause of the weight gain, and this can certainly happen.[30] But the
significant rise in diagnoses of low testosterone suggests something
else is occurring (unless you espouse the idea that men have spontaneously become "less manly"). Thus, before we conclude that men have,
within a generation, evolved to spontaneously develop low testosterone and become obese and infertile, it's worthwhile to explore the
process in reverse—to consider that poor metabolic health is actually
preceding and causing the reduced testosterone production.

Men with higher body fat tend to have less testosterone,[31] and testosterone levels increase as a man loses weight.[32] Of course, insulin is
highly relevant in these changes, though it can be hard to distinguish
insulin's direct effect from a potential independent effect of simply
having too much adipose (fat) tissue. The results of several studies[33]
have confirmed that insulin, independent of body fat, directly inhibits testosterone production; more insulin leads to lower testosterone.

THE OVARY IN THE ADIPOSE

Ovaries in women, unlike testes in men, produce relatively fewer androgens. Rather, ovaries are equipped with high levels of aromatase—as we
learned on page 42, that's the very busy enzyme that changes male hormones (androgens) to female hormones (estrogens). (This also happens in the testes, just not as much.)

Remarkably, aromatase also exists in fat tissue.[34] Yes, men: your fat
tissue is acting like an ovary. More precisely, excess fat tissue increases
circulating estrogens in both men and women. (So, if your doctor tells
you you're "low T," don't blame your testes for what your fat did!)

Sperm Production

While perhaps not as complex as ovulation, sperm production never-theless requires the involvement of several hormones, including some from the brain, and testosterone and even estrogens from the testes. Disruptions in the normal production of these hormones can result in the failure to produce sufficient or healthy sperm. If testosterone is below normal levels, sperm production cannot occur.[35]

Erectile Dysfunction

Men with insulin resistance have an increased risk of erectile dysfunction,[36] and erectile dysfunction gets worse as insulin resistance gets more severe.[37] Indeed, the relationship is so tight that erectile dys-function could be one of the earliest signs of insulin resistance, with scientists recently stating in a research article that "insulin resistance may be the underlying pathogenesis of ED in young patients without well-known etiology."[38] In other words, if a seemingly healthy young man has erectile dysfunction, insulin resistance could very well be the cause. But to appreciate this connection, we need to revisit the power-ful influence insulin wields on blood vessels.

Erectile dysfunction typically stems from a problem of blood ves-sel regulation—blood vessels must dilate dramatically to develop and sustain an erection. This process requires the production and actions of NO.[39] As we discussed in chapter two, as endothelial cells (the cells that line the walls of the blood vessels) become insulin resistant, they produce less nitric oxide, which deprives the blood vessels of a strong dilating signal.

If a woman's fertility is like an orchestra, a man's fertility is like a barbershop quartet—fewer parts, but each one essential. The com-plication for men is that fertility requires both physical (i.e., erection) *and* hormonal (i.e., sperm production) processes. In both instances, insulin sings the lead and keeps the other characters on key.

Insulin and Puberty

The transition from childhood to adulthood is a period of intense change—notoriously, an intense hormonal change. This all usually starts in the brain with the release of gonadotropin-releasing hormone

(GnRH). GnRH sends a signal to adolescent ovaries and testes to induce higher levels of estrogens and androgens that, in turn, lead to the development of secondary sex characteristics—facial hair and voice changes in boys, selective increases in fat and wider hips in girls, and substantial growth in both.

This period of rapid growth requires tremendous energy. And because hormones dictate energy use within the body, puberty is intimately linked, not only with obvious physical changes, but also with changes in our metabolic function.

To understand how metabolism ties in to puberty, we need to understand the role of yet another hormone, leptin. Leptin is a metabolic hormone secreted from fat tissue; the more fat tissue you have, the more leptin you'll usually have circulating in your blood. You might have heard of leptin as a hormone that sends an "I'm full" signal to the brain, letting the body know when it's eaten enough. Leptin does much more, including telling the brain there is sufficient body fat to sexually develop. Essentially, leptin increases the production of GnRH from the brain, thereby driving puberty. This effect is so strong that, in mice, leptin injections alone are sufficient to induce puberty.[40]

At first glance, the topic of puberty has plenty to do with other hormones but not much to do with insulin. However, insulin and leptin are highly related and influence each other. As insulin rises, it stimulates leptin production from fat cells, which then activates precursor sex hormone production in the brain, then the gonads. Because insulin has a part to play here, it means our metabolic health and our nutrition have a strong influence on when puberty begins.

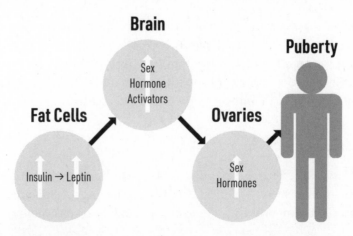

Overnutrition and Early Puberty

Various factors determine when puberty will begin. Some of those factors, such as family history,[41] are expected, while others are unexpected—for example, it might surprise you that girls with supportive parental relationships are likely to start puberty later than girls who don't.[42] One of the strongest determinants of when puberty will start is a person's nutrition and body fat mass.[43] (Perhaps because women bear the metabolic burden in reproduction, having to carry the developing baby and feed the newborn, puberty in girls appears to be much more sensitive to metabolic and nutrition status than puberty in boys.)

In recent years, a global shift has occurred in nutrition. Whereas we were once concerned with people around the world not having enough food, the problem of people eating too much food is now more common. Importantly, much of the food we're overeating comes in the form of refined and insulin-spiking carbohydrates, such as sugar.[44] Parallel with this shift in nutrition and lifestyle is an equally dramatic increase in blood insulin levels.[45]

As highlighted earlier, insulin drives body fat growth—as insulin climbs, it promotes fat cell development and growth, and prevents the breakdown of fat stored in these cells. As fat cells expand, they produce and secrete more leptin into the blood. The relationship between leptin and insulin becomes particularly important in the context of puberty and, especially, the early onset of puberty, known as precocious puberty. The result is that over the decades, the global overeating crisis, with its changes in insulin and leptin, has had stark effects on puberty.

Current standards mark a normal onset for puberty to be from around eight to 12 years old in girls and nine to 14 years old in boys. However, our current lifestyle is very different than in earlier generations, and perhaps in all of human history. To put this in perspective, the average onset of puberty in the mid-1800s was around 16 years for girls. This dropped to around 14 in the early 1900s, then to 13 and 12 in the mid- and late 1900s, respectively. Now the average age is under 10 years old—a difference in puberty onset of almost seven years!

The connection between obesity and precocious puberty is strong enough to quantify; every one-unit increase in body mass index (BMI; a rough indicator of body fat) between the ages of two to eight is associated with a roughly one-month-earlier onset of puberty.[46] In other words, if a young girl's BMI increases five points above average (a very possible change) during this age range, she can expect puberty to start a half year earlier than what would be normal for her.

There has been speculation as to the cause of these changes. Many theories center around girls' exposure to estrogen-like molecules found in detergents and plastics. While this might have an influence, the role of insulin resistance and hyperinsulinemia is irrefutable. Again, excess insulin drives excess leptin production, which leads to early puberty. Medical intervention aimed at increasing insulin sensitivity (discussed in depth later), with a subsequent reduction in insulin and leptin, slows the age of puberty onset and progression to normal.[47]

UNDERNUTRITION AND PUBERTY

Though much less common, it's worthwhile to highlight undernutrition and puberty. If a child is undernourished, the effect on puberty depends on *when* the lack of sufficient food occurred.

In one scenario, if a child is born under her ideal body weight, she will commonly catch up to her peers in the first few years of life, and, within the next few years, exceed them in body fat gain. Because of this, children that are born underweight usually experience puberty at the same time as their peers, though they may also start earlier than normal[48]; this is especially true for girls. Remember, below-average birthweight increases the risk of developing insulin resistance.[49] So, in these children who are born relatively undernourished, as body fat catches up to normal, then surpasses it, insulin starts relatively lower in life, then increases in the ensuing years with the progression of insulin resistance. The higher insulin levels increase leptin levels and make it more likely that puberty will start early.

The second scenario involves a child who experiences undernutrition in childhood preceding puberty but had a normal birthweight. This child's diet or lifestyle is such that insulin is very low, which results in very little body fat. This, in turn, results in insufficient leptin production,[50] leading to delayed puberty. A prime example of this is the young female gymnast who undertakes strict training and diet to maximize her performance by reducing body fat and increasing muscle mass.

In these elite gymnasts, delayed puberty is very common.[51] A second example of delayed puberty with undernutrition is the individual with anorexia nervosa, a state of self-imposed starvation. Puberty is usually delayed in this state, and, in some instances, physical sexual development may be permanently hindered, even if nutrition later becomes sufficient (e.g., reduced breast development).[52]

Reproduction is a demanding process, and the body wants to ensure things are working right, including metabolic function, before worrying about the next generation. Insulin, the king of all metabolic hormones, is a strong indicator of metabolic status in the body—and high insulin rings a warning bell. From the brain to the ovaries and testes, insulin either facilitates or frustrates reproduction. Normal insulin, reflecting good metabolic health, promotes normal fertility.

As frustrating as fertility issues can be, they rarely fall within the realm of "scary," which is where the next health complication resides. As different as fertility and cancer are, they do have one thing in common—to varying degrees, they're both influenced by insulin.

CHAPTER 5

Cancer

CANCER IS THE SECOND-LEADING CAUSE OF DEATH in the United States, although it's making a strong play to overtake heart disease as killer number one.[1] Cancers can affect any organ. Breast and prostate cancers are the most common in women and men, respectively, and lung cancer is the deadliest. Despite over $160 billion being spent per year to cure cancer in the US, with a global economic burden of roughly $1.2 trillion, ever more people are dying. Clearly, this investment isn't paying off.

Cancers have different possible causes. While the general consensus is that cancer results from genetic mutations or gene damage, increasing evidence challenges this conclusion. Perhaps cancer isn't a disease of genetics, but rather of metabolism. Though it's controversial, the metabolic paradigm isn't without significant supporting data, some of which began a century ago (discussed more hereafter).[2]

Regardless of its specific cause, cancer is a disease of cellular growth; certain cells begin to multiply uncontrollably. And insulin resistance is part of this equation because it pushes cancer cells to grow faster. With insulin resistance, we have a perfect storm involving two primary ingredients on which cancer cells thrive.

First, cancer cells seem to have a sweet tooth—they love glucose.[3] Now, normally, our cells are awash in a constant supply of nutrients. Because our bodies don't want all our cells to proliferate unchecked, we have natural control systems in place—healthy cells don't take in nutrients unless they're specifically told to do so by substances called growth factors. When they get the signal, normal cells take in nutrients and rely on enzymes to burn them, thereby releasing energy that becomes our body's fuel. This energy-creation process takes place inside our cells' mitochondria. However, cancer cells actually rewire their metabolism to get their energy a different way. Almost 100 years ago, the German physician and scientist Otto Heinrich Warburg discovered that cancer cells have an almost total reliance on glucose as their primary metabolic fuel. Moreover, Warburg's research indicated that, instead of using their mitochondria to break down the glucose, they do so outside the mitochondria, without the need of oxygen (the technical term for this is anaerobic glycolysis). We now refer to this phenomenon as the "Warburg effect." This critical deviation from the norm allows cancer cells to grow rapidly everywhere in the body, including locations that might not have adequate blood flow (and, therefore, not enough oxygen).

Second, as you know by now, with insulin resistance, blood insulin levels are elevated. When you appreciate that one of insulin's main actions is to cause cells to grow, you can easily appreciate the predicament. Insulin's anabolic effects can also work to increase the growth of cancer cells, especially if the cancer cell has made itself more sensitive to insulin than a normal cell. Thus, while the high blood insulin is sending signals for fat cells to grow, any cancer cells that have mutated to be more sensitive to insulin are growing far more rapidly than normal thanks to this boost from insulin.

To further emphasize insulin's relevance in cancer, one of the most studied aspects of cancer is something called the insulin-like growth factor-1. This protein, like insulin, promotes general growth in the body. That's usually a good thing, but it is also a common feature of many cancers.[4]

The combination of these two signals, glucose and insulin, is essential to understanding why people with hyperinsulinemia—whether they are lean or fat—have roughly double the likelihood of dying from cancer.[5] What's worse is that breast, prostate, and colorectal cancers have a stronger relevance to insulin resistance.

Breast Cancer

The cancer perhaps most commonly linked to insulin resistance is breast cancer, which is also the most common cancer in US women (though very rarely—less than 1% of cases—men can also develop breast cancer). The fact that it's *not* the most common worldwide highlights the importance of environment in so many diseases, including cancers. And insulin resistance has a very strong connection to our environment—we'll explore that in depth in Part II.

Women with the highest fasting insulin levels (that is, women with insulin resistance) are those with the worst breast cancer outcomes.[6] Remember, insulin tells cells, including cancer cells, to grow. But the increased insulin alone may account for only part of the insulin–breast cancer connection. The average breast cancer tumor has over six times more insulin receptors than noncancerous breast tissue.[7] Six times more! That means this malignant tissue is six times more responsive to insulin and its growth signals than normal tissues.

Ultimately, the connection between insulin resistance and breast cancer has been so consistently observed over the years that when trials began treating breast cancer patients with insulin-sensitizing medications, it wasn't surprising to see an improvement in the disease.[8] Essentially, the researchers found that controlling insulin resistance helped control the breast cancer.

A related connection is the role of fat tissue itself. We'll spend two chapters exploring the complicated relationship between insulin resistance and obesity, and we have previously highlighted how excess body fat increases circulating estrogens (see "The Ovary in the Adipose" on page 44). Breast tissue is sensitive to estrogens—estrogens send a growth signal to breast tissue. When this happens excessively, such as is the case with obesity, the breast tissue is more likely to grow excessively, increasing the risk of developing breast cancer.[9]

Prostate Cancer

Prostate cancer is the most common cancer in men in the United States, and it becomes increasingly common in men as they age. And prostate cancer, too, has a strong connection with insulin resistance.

Like the breast, the prostate is a highly hormone-sensitive tissue; it will grow or shrink based on hormone signals. While testosterone is the main hormone signal, insulin also plays a role. Before a man is worried about prostate cancer, he's worried about his prostate just getting too big—a condition called benign prostatic hyperplasia. This is a very common event in men as they age, usually causing difficulty in urinating (the enlarged/growing prostate blocks the exit of urine from the bladder). A man with insulin resistance is about two to three times more likely to have an enlarged prostate compared with an insulin-sensitive man.[10] So, high insulin means low flow.

Men with a high degree of insulin resistance may be upwards of 250% more likely to develop prostate cancer compared with insulin-sensitive men of the same age, race, and body weight.[11] In fact, prostate cancer and insulin resistance occur together so often that some scientists have questioned whether prostate cancer might be an additional eventual *symptom* of insulin resistance.[12] Critically, an analysis of 500 men found that insulin (but not glucose) was positively associated with prostate cancer risk.[13]

But the insulin–prostate connection doesn't end with elevated insulin levels in the blood. Similar to breast cancer, a fairly common feature with prostate tumors both malignant and benign, is the presence of excess insulin receptors.[14] So once again, the excess blood insulin and the increased number of insulin receptors in the prostate combine to create a powerful "growth" signal, stimulating the prostate to grow beyond its normal limitations.

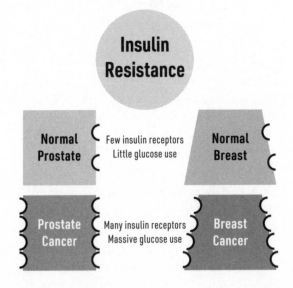

Colorectal Cancer

Insulin resistance is associated with increased risk of developing cancer in the lower part of the digestive tract, including the colon and rectum; it also makes colorectal cancer more lethal.[15] Indeed, colon cancer patients with insulin resistance are roughly *three times* more likely to die from the cancer, compared with patients who do not have insulin resistance. The hyperinsulinemia that invariably accompanies (causes) insulin resistance may be the main driver of colon cancer development.[16]

Too much insulin has been shown to increase the number of cells of the outermost (mucosal) layer of the intestines.[17] This might seem like a good thing, but when we consider that cancer is a problem wherein cells are excessively growing and proliferating, it's perhaps not so benign.

Cancer is a terrifying disease, partly due to its seeming randomness; healthy people who "do everything right" can still get cancer, while some lifelong smokers get nothing. Undoubtedly, there are variables outside of our control—age and genetics, for example. Thus, emphasizing the controllable variables, such as our environment and the food we eat, is the most rational strategy to mitigate our cancer risk and improve our outcome if we do get it. There is no single most relevant player with cancer, but insulin resistance clearly plays one of the leading roles. Thankfully, as we will see, it's one we can do something about.

Now that we've covered the heavy topic of cancer, it's time to discuss the "filling"—all the parts of our bodies that make up our ability to move and work. Even these, as you'll see, are susceptible to changes in insulin.

CHAPTER 6

Aging, the Skin, Muscles, and Bones

A̲T MIDDLE AGE, I've come to a personal realization: I'm not what I used to be. Sure, I'm wiser, but my body doesn't move or look how it used to. I suspect you may have had the same realization. As we grow older, our bodies undergo major changes: our skin becomes looser and dryer, our muscles grow weak, our bones may become porous and brittle. We don't fully understand the mechanisms that explain how we age, but because none of us is immune, we're understandably very curious about it.

At its simplest, aging is the sum consequence of our cells losing the ability to replenish themselves, which translates to our organs and, ultimately, our entire body not working like it once did. In our exhaustive study of aging, many theories have been proposed to explain why we age, each with evidence to support it. Some prominent theories include inherent genetic limitations that cap the number of times a cell can replicate. Others are based on the idea that harmful environmental factors lead to cellular damage, such as oxidative stress or inflammation. But a newer theory implicates insulin resistance as a cause for aging, and the evidence is compelling.

Experiments in several organisms, including yeast, worms, flies, and mice, provide conclusive evidence that insulin resistance is connected to longevity. In these organisms, slowing down insulin action—either by reducing insulin levels or by selectively blocking its action—results in the insect or animal living up to 50% longer than normal.[1] Importantly, this doesn't just include organisms with a genetic change in insulin signaling, but even those that have simply been given a diet that keeps insulin low![2] However, these findings may not apply to humans.

AGING AND THE LOW-CALORIE CONTROVERSY

Decades ago, advocates of the "damage theory" of aging posited that a calorie-restricted diet would extend an individual's lifespan. The most conclusive studies on this used monkeys, which are among humans' closest animal relatives. Enthusiasm for this theory exploded when, in 2009, scientists found that calorie restriction indeed resulted in an average extension of life.[3] However, it was later revealed that calorie-restricted animals that died from causes "other than aging," such as infections, were not included in the study. When these monkeys were included, there was no difference in average lifespan. The theory took another hit when another similar study in monkeys in 2012 found no lifespan benefit.[4]

It would be foolish to attempt to assign all of aging's problems or its root cause *entirely* to insulin resistance. Still, one critical fact that supports this theory is that the longest-living humans are also the most insulin sensitive—true even after controlling for seemingly obvious variables, including body mass and sex.[5] Further, people who have a particular variation in insulin-related genes are more likely to live longer than those without the variation.[6] And current research supports the idea that insulin-sensitizing medications may slow aging.

While the actual process of growing old is a mix of several factors, almost every feature of aging, including skin changes, reduced muscle mass, bone loss, and more, is a consequence of insulin resistance.

Insulin Resistance and the Skin

Skin is composed of many different types of cells, each with a distinct function. The skin is also surprisingly insulin responsive. You may have heard that diabetes causes skin issues—people who have diabetes tend to have extremely dry, itchy skin; are prone to frequent skin infections; and can have trouble healing wounds. While these complaints generally stem from high blood glucose and/or poor circulation, there are in fact several skin pathologies related to changes in insulin. Many of them can develop well before adulthood.

Acanthosis Nigricans

Acanthosis nigricans can be the first sign that someone has insulin resistance. The condition involves overactive melanocytes. These are cells embedded in the skin that create a molecule called melanin—the stuff that provides the pigment or tone of the skin. Darker skin has more melanin, and lighter skin has less.

Like all cells of the body, melanocytes are sensitive to insulin; high blood insulin makes the melanocytes overactive, ultimately increasing melanin production to the degree that the skin takes a darker-than-normal tone.[7] However, this isn't an alternative for a fake tan! This darkening occurs most often where the skin rubs together, such as the neck, armpits, and groin, but it can also appear as large patches anywhere on the trunk, arms, legs, or face. These pigment changes are usually noticeable on all skin colors, though they may be more obvious on individuals with lighter complexions. (Importantly, dark patches in the mouth are a potential sign of a melanoma—a cancer of the melanocytes.)

Anyone with insulin resistance, including people who are obese or have type 2 diabetes, is more likely to see the skin changes of acanthosis nigricans. Moreover, it can develop at any age, affecting even insulin-resistant children.

Skin Tags

Have you ever wondered about those small little flaps of skin you might have or have seen on others? Known formally as "acrochorda" and informally as "skin tags," these little bumps are frequently seen with acanthosis nigricans and, hence, usually occur in the same distinct areas (neck, armpits, groin). People with insulin resistance are much more likely to develop skin tags compared with insulin-sensitive counterparts.[8] The connection between insulin resistance and skin tags is likely a result of hyperinsulinemia stimulating the growth and division of keratinocytes—a cell that provides structure to the skin.

Psoriasis

Psoriasis is a chronic inflammatory skin disease, usually manifesting as psoriasis vulgaris—well-defined sections of reddish or pinkish skin covered by white or silvery scales. Psoriasis often develops on the elbows and knees, scalp, or midsection. It can develop at any age, though most often between adolescence and age 35.

We don't know exactly what causes psoriasis, though it seems that the immune system and genetics are involved. That said, there's an insulin connection. People with psoriasis are significantly more likely to have metabolic complications, such as insulin resistance.[9] In fact, the connection is sufficiently strong that people with psoriasis are almost three times more likely than normal to be insulin resistant.[10]

Acne

While often prominent during teenage years, acne, which can occur throughout adulthood, is typified by excessive comedones (blackheads or whiteheads) on the face, neck, back, or elsewhere. Whether they're lean or overweight, people with acne have higher fasting levels of insulin in the blood compared with people without acne. One study looked at the connection between insulin resistance and acne by giving young men with and without acne a glucose solution to drink. Remarkably, insulin levels spiked over four times higher in overweight participants with acne and more than doubled in lean ones with acne.[11]

So much of what we've discussed is devoted to highlighting the serious and potentially life-threatening consequences of insulin resistance. While those deserve attention, they're also hard to see—you can't see plaques developing in your brain or your blood pressure climbing, but you can see changes in your skin.

INSULIN RESISTANCE AND HEARING LOSS

Hearing loss and bouts of vertigo are often considered regrettable but unavoidable consequences of aging. Perhaps it's not our age causing them, but the metabolic disruption that's accumulated as we grow older.

Almost everyone loses some hearing with age; this is known as presbycusis. In fact, presbycusis is so common it's considered the number one communicative disorder with aging. Even when controlling for weight and age, if a person is insulin resistant, inner ear function is significantly compromised.[12] In particular, the greater the insulin resistance, the greater difficulty in hearing lower tones.

Another common ear disorder is Ménière's disease. Believed to be a problem of fluid accumulation in the inner ear, Ménière's disease can cause vertigo, ringing in your ear (tinnitus), and hearing loss. The connection between Ménière's disease and insulin resistance is strong; one study found that 76% of patients with Ménière's were also insulin resistant.[13] Other data reveal that up to 92% of people with tinnitus have hyperinsulinemia![14] Thus, it's very likely that a person suffering with ringing in the ears is somewhere on the spectrum of insulin resistance. Indeed, Dr. William Updegraff, a prominent otolaryngologist, boldly claimed, after first exploring this connection over 40 years ago, "The most common—and most overlooked—cause of vertigo is a disorder of glucose metabolism."[15]

Insulin and Muscle Function

In the average middle-aged person, muscle accounts for roughly 25%–30% of body mass, which makes it the largest insulin-sensitive tissue in the body. Muscle is also very responsive to insulin, which elicits several important effects, such as promoting muscle growth and maintenance and regulating protein metabolism. And in the context of insulin resistance, muscle is very important—how much of it we have and how insulin sensitive it is, is vital in determining how insulin sensitive our entire body is. This is largely a function of muscle's ability to take up glucose from the blood in response to insulin; as glucose drops, insulin returns to baseline. As the amount of muscle increases or decreases, insulin sensitivity changes accordingly.[16] Naturally, this means if we have more muscle, we have more "room" to deposit glucose and remove it from the blood, which helps keep insulin low and maintain a higher degree of insulin sensitivity.

With insulin resistance, the muscle is approximately half as insulin sensitive as it should be[17]—and muscle is usually one of the first tissues to become insulin resistant. Insulin resistance compromises healthy muscle function, potentially contributing to muscle loss, reduced muscle capacity, and decreased performance.

Muscle Loss

Sarcopenia is the term for muscle loss that accompanies aging; we lose roughly 1% of our muscle each year after middle age.[18]

Of course, losing muscle is a somewhat normal part of aging, stemming from changes in several hormones, including growth hormone and androgens. But as a muscle becomes resistant to the effects of insulin, this includes a resistance to insulin's anabolic effects, and the muscle loses a potent growth signal.

To maintain or grow muscle, the muscle must produce enough cellular protein to compensate for any protein loss. This phenomenon is referred to as protein turnover, and it can be negative (the muscle is losing more protein than it's building), neutral (protein loss is matched by protein building), or positive (the muscle is building more protein than it's losing). Insulin stimulates muscle protein creation while preventing muscle protein degradation, helping a muscle be in neutral, if not positive, protein turnover. But all of this is contingent, of course, on the muscle sensing and responding to insulin. People with insulin resistance, outside of the effects of aging, have a relative increase in muscle protein breakdown compared with insulin-sensitive people of the same age.[19] In other words, if you're insulin resistant, you'll have a harder time promoting muscle growth or even maintaining muscle mass.

INSULIN AND BODY BUILDERS: A LOVE STORY

Competitive (and not-so-competitive) bodybuilders, like any athlete, are interested in any strategy that gives them an advantage. Sometimes this includes using illicit substances like anabolic steroids and human growth hormone; some may turn to seemingly benign hormones like insulin. Its ability to stimulate skeletal muscle growth is real, but (as

I hope is clear by now!), when chronically elevated, insulin is far from benign. An informed user would need to consider the effects other than muscle growth, including insulin resistance, high blood cholesterol, high blood pressure, dementia, and so on. But hey! At least you'd have big muscles . . . that is, of course, until the progressive insulin resistance makes them ever-more difficult to maintain.

Fibromyalgia

Fibromyalgia is one of the most common generalized pain disorders. In response to the question, "How do you feel?" someone with fibromyalgia can only reply "I just ache." The widespread muscle pain is often accompanied by fatigue, memory problems, and mood issues. In addition to the frustration of these symptoms, many people with fibromyalgia never get an explanation for the cause of their pain; some first experience it after a surgery, infection, or physical trauma, but in other cases, there's no obvious trigger. However, very recent findings suggest that insulin resistance could be a cause. In "Is Insulin Resistance the Cause of Fibromyalgia: A Preliminary Report," researchers revealed that people with fibromyalgia are significantly more likely to struggle with insulin and glucose control.[20]

Clearly, insulin resistance can wreak havoc for our muscles; insulin plays a major role in keeping them healthy and strong. Of course, our muscles would be useless without a rigid structure to allow movement; that structure is provided by our bones and joints.

Insulin and the Bones and Joints

Our bones do much more than provide structure, allowing us to stand and move. They also protect our organs, store minerals, and produce our red and white blood cells. Bones, like most tissues, regularly change. Like a muscle, with its high protein need, proper bone health requires bone matrix turnover: the bone is constantly degrading and rebuilding its contents, and calcium and other minerals are being added to and taken from the bone. This involves the actions of two predominant cells: osteoblasts, which strengthen and create new bone to replace old bone, and osteoclasts, which degrade old bone. Together, these two cell types ensure we have sufficient and healthy bone mass.

Bone insulin signaling hasn't received nearly as much attention as muscle insulin signaling; thus not as much is known about bone insulin resistance. However, we're starting to learn more, and it's clear that insulin helps maintain bone mass. The cooperative effort between osteoblasts and osteoclasts functions, at least partly, because of the disparate effect insulin has on each. Whereas insulin stimulates osteoblast activity,[21] promoting bone growth, it inhibits osteoclast action,[22] reducing bone degradation. Altogether, insulin increases bone by supporting growth and preventing loss.

CAN BONES DETERMINE INSULIN SENSITIVITY?

In addition to their essential bone-building role, osteoblasts also secrete a hormone called osteocalcin. In a study of mice, osteocalcin injections improved insulin resistance and prevented type 2 diabetes onset.[23] Interestingly, the relationship persists in humans—people with low levels of osteocalcin are much more likely to be insulin resistant, and vice versa.[24] The relevance of this finding may be the role that vitamin D plays; osteoblasts require vitamin D to produce osteocalcin.[25] Indeed, this may explain how vitamin D is so commonly linked to improving insulin sensitivity; a 2019 study in boys found that insulin resistance was tightly linked with compromised bone growth during adolescence.[26]

Reduced Bone Mass

Many of us have heard of osteoporosis, a state wherein the bones are thin and weak. Along the way to osteoporosis, we would experience osteopenia; this is when the bones are thinner and weaker than normal but not yet to the point of osteoporosis.

Researchers exploring the effect of insulin resistance on bone health have to grapple with the complication of body weight. Whether they are heavier from fat or from muscle, bigger bodies have bigger bones; insulin resistance is associated with more body fat.[27]

Considerable evidence reveals that while people with insulin resistance may have normal (or even greater than normal) bone mass, which could be a result of moving around a heavier body, they paradoxically have reduced bone strength and are much more likely to have fractures.[28] Still, there's not a consensus among researchers regarding what happens to bone health with insulin resistance. Several reports indicate contrasting findings,[29] though some of this confusion may be a result of various drugs the insulin-resistant individual is taking.[30]

More than just moving us around, bone mass has important implications for those facing life-threatening diseases requiring drastic, life-changing procedures. In particular, people with leukemia, a cancer of blood cells, require a bone marrow transplant, which means they have had their bones filled with a population of someone else's cells. A group of researchers wanted to understand the difference between people who lose bone mass and those who don't during the course of this procedure. Interestingly, they found that patients who are insulin resistant are much more likely to experience a reduction in bone mass when compared with insulin-sensitive individuals. In fact, insulin resistance was the only variable that separated the two groups.[31]

Osteoarthritis

While good bone health is readily acknowledged as necessary for high quality of life, bones are of little use without healthy joints to move them. Osteoarthritis, or the loss of joint cartilage, was once considered a disease of excessive wear and tear. Because it's a common occurrence in obesity, many physicians assumed it was a simple consequence of joints carrying around too much weight for too long. However, it is increasingly considered a metabolic disease. Like so many tissues, even our joints are sensitive to metabolic signals, including insulin. Out of a broad range of overweight individuals researchers studied, those with osteoarthritis were most likely to have the highest insulin levels.[32]

An essential component of the joint is the cartilage: the smooth, flexible connective tissue lining the ends of the bones that articulate a joint. The main cells in cartilage are called chondrocytes and, of course, they are insulin responsive. They are responsible for creating and maintaining the cartilage lining, known as a matrix; this is made largely of collagen and substances that the chondrocytes need glucose to create. And, the chondrocytes need insulin to take in that glucose[33]; an insulin-resistant chondrocyte can't maintain that matrix, and, ultimately, the cartilage weakens.

Another essential component of a joint, beyond its lining, is the "grease" for the joint—synovial fluid. Synovial fluid is made from specialized cells called synoviocytes, which, just like the chondrocytes, play an essential role in helping the joint work well. When synoviocytes are exposed to high levels of insulin, they experience an invasion of immune cells that ramp up inflammation in the joint and reduce synovial fluid production.[34] Without this grease, the gears just grind.

Osteoarthritis shouldn't be confused with rheumatoid arthritis, which is a chronic inflammatory joint disease. Likely because of the inflammation it creates, rheumatoid arthritis increases the likelihood of developing insulin resistance (we'll discuss the role of inflammation in insulin resistance in Part II). In fact, the severity and activity of the disease can wax and wane over time, and the accompanying insulin resistance similarly will become more or less severe.[35]

FIXING ONE PROBLEM BUT CAUSING ANOTHER

Many people with joint pains take glucosamine in some form, which *may* improve joint health and reduce joint pain, though evidence is equivocal.[36] However, while it *may* improve your joints, the glucosamine is very likely making you more insulin resistant.[37] The evidence isn't equivocal at all—across humans and rodents, glucosamine makes a body less insulin sensitive.

Gout

Gout is a type of inflammatory joint disease where the joint accumulates uric acid crystals and the inflammation that accompanies them. The joints most commonly affected are those in your limbs, including your feet (especially the big toe), ankles, fingers, and wrists.

Uric acid is normally excreted by the kidneys into the urine (as the name suggests) and eliminated from the body. However, insulin resistance changes this process, making the kidneys accrue uric acid rather than excrete it.[38] Uric acid then builds up in the blood and settles in the joints just mentioned, initiating a local inflammatory reaction that causes the redness and swelling typical of gout.

Our muscles, bones, and skin have a common theme—they "connect" the body, allowing it to act as one unit. This connective tissue requires insulin's actions to maintain its strength and integrity, though this isn't unique to these bulky (muscle and bone) and stretchy (skin) tissues. Now that we looked at the tissues that cover and move us, let's dive back into the body to see how insulin resistance alters the tissues that nourish and clean us.

CHAPTER 7

Gastrointestinal and Kidney Health

OUR INTESTINES AND KIDNEYS are vital to life and share the burden of keeping our bodies clean—they work to block harmful substances from entering or staying in our systems and push them from the body. Tragically, they're both highly susceptible to insulin resistance. A shocking number (about 63%) of people with insulin resistance (type 2 diabetes) experience gastrointestinal issues. It's also the leading cause of kidney failure. So our response to insulin is closely tied to our gastrointestinal and kidney health; if we expect these organs to work their best, we need to keep insulin in control.

Insulin and Digestion

The gastrointestinal (GI) tract includes everything from mouth to anus, as well as multiple associated organs, such as the liver, gallbladder, and pancreas. All of these players work together to digest foods and absorb the nutrients from the gut into the blood. This process involves multiple distinct steps: we chew and swallow our food (while enzymes in our saliva begin the digestive process), food moves through the intestines, certain glands secrete digestive substances into the intestines, these substances break down the food into smaller molecules, and then these smaller molecules move through the intestinal cells and into the blood. Each step requires the previous step to work in concert. And insulin resistance can create problems with all of them.

Reflux Esophagitis

To digest foods, the stomach produces a highly acidic juice. The stomach can handle this acid because it is lined with thick protective mucus, but the esophagus can't withstand it, so a ring of muscles called the lower esophageal sphincter closes off the esophagus from the stomach. However, sometimes stomach contents are still able to splash up (or reflux) into the esophagus. Because the esophagus has no protection from the highly acidic mix, the lower esophagus can develop ulcers as a result.

Almost half (about 40%) of all American adults experience frequent heartburn, the common symptom of reflux.[1] When we recall that over half of American adults are insulin resistant, it's not surprising to learn that metabolic syndrome is highly related to reflux esophagitis and to its chronic cousin, gastroesophageal reflux disease.[2] In particular, two key symptoms of metabolic syndrome are linked here: visceral obesity and insulin resistance. The connection with visceral obesity may be easier to grasp: having more fat in the central region may compress the surrounding tissues, including the stomach. That would increase stomach pressure and relax the lower esophageal sphincter. As I have mentioned at various points, and as we'll see in more detail in the next chapter, insulin resistance can lead to visceral obesity. But—and this is critical—although visceral obesity may be the obvious culprit for reflux, it's not acting on its own. In scrutinizing numerous lifestyle variables, physicians in Taiwan found that insulin resistance, independent of visceral obesity, blood pressure, or other variables, increases the risk of developing reflux by approximately 15%; to put it plainly, the subjects' reflux got worse as their insulin resistance got worse.[3]

Over time, the lower end of the esophagus begins to defend itself from acid reflux by changing the outermost layer of cells into a more robust lining that resembles the lining of the intestines. This is a condition called Barrett's esophagus, which is more prevalent with insulin resistance.[4] Alone, Barrett's esophagus may not be a serious or life-threatening condition, though it can lead to uncomfortable and/or painful swallowing. However, once cells start changing, they may continue to change, potentially becoming malignant. Thus, the real concern with Barrett's esophagus is the potential that it might develop into esophageal cancer.[5]

Gastroparesis

Let's continue our journey along the GI tract. To push the food we've eaten through the intestines and eventually out of the body, the intestines steadily contract and relax in a pattern of involuntary transport called peristalsis. Gastroparesis is a potentially serious complication wherein the intestines, and usually the stomach, are paralyzed and unable to move food onward. This results in the food lingering and potentially condensing into a hard mass called a bezoar that can block narrow passages as it moves, slowly and painfully, through the intestines.

Diabetes is a prominent cause of gastroparesis. In people with diabetes, the condition is thought to stem from the damage that can happen to specific nerves, known as neuropathy.[6] In this instance, the nerve that controls the stomach, the vagus nerve, becomes damaged and thus is less able to induce stomach contractions and peristalsis. This nerve damage is likely a consequence of the excess blood glucose that typifies diabetes, but even insulin alone has an effect. One study gave its participants infusions of insulin to create an artificial hyperinsulinemia, like what would accompany insulin resistance, and the movement of food through their intestines was slowed by almost 40%.[7]

THE DOWN SIDE OF PUSHING DOWN GLUCOSE

Interestingly, the gut and kidneys are common "sites of attack" when it comes to controlling glucose in the body, which affects insulin. Because blood insulin is so yoked to blood glucose (i.e., rising glucose pushes up insulin), it's interesting to note two classes of drugs that try to control glucose and insulin. One strategy works in the gut by turning off glucose digestion (e.g., alpha-glucosidase inhibitors), forcing the glucose to stay in the gut unchanged, thus *preventing* it from entering the blood. Unfortunately, the undigested glucose results in something called "osmotic diarrhea,"[8] which is as pleasant as it sounds. The second strategy pushes the glucose *out* of the blood by forcing the kidneys to dump blood glucose into the urine at artificially high levels. Tragically, by pushing glucose into the urinary tract, the ever-present bacteria there thrive in the midst of all that glucose, increasing one's rate of urinary tract infection.[9] So, whether moving glucose into the body or pushing glucose out of the body, the digestive and urinary tracts are relevant to controlling glucose and insulin.

Of course, the intestines can't really fulfill their role without some help. Acting alone, the intestines are basically a tube through which food and eventual waste moves through us—so they can only transport matter and absorb nutrients and water. For proper digestion to occur before absorption, the intestines rely on several organs, which we'll explore now.

Insulin and the Liver

If we were to rate the organs of the body by how many physiological processes they handle, the liver would be number one. The liver is essential for removing toxins from the blood, clearing old blood cells, storing vitamins, nutrient metabolism (e.g., handling of fats, proteins, and carbohydrates), and much more. This widespread involvement in so many critical processes may be partly why the liver has been such a focus of medical, even cultural, attention. In Persian cultures, particularly in Iran, a common term of endearment is to refer to a special someone as *jigar tala* or "golden liver!"

People likely can't develop whole-body insulin resistance without the liver being insulin resistant, and the liver may be one of the first organs to do so.[10] When a healthy liver senses insulin in the blood, it will take in glucose—not to use right away, but rather to store as backup energy for the body. It converts some to a substance called glycogen, which is just several glucose molecules linked together, and some to fat. This lowers the amount of glucose in the blood, which helps lower insulin. However, once insulin resistant, the liver begins to create a uniquely pathogenic situation, increasing blood glucose and fats, as well as potentially altering LDL cholesterol size (which, as we discussed earlier, can increase the risk of blood vessels becoming hard and narrow—see pages 18–22).[11]

Normally, glycogen is held for reserve energy in our liver and muscles. When the body senses that energy is needed—in response to low blood glucose or stress or to help our digestion—the glycogen is converted back into glucose and released into the bloodstream. With insulin resistance, insulin no longer tells the liver to take in and store that glucose as glycogen. In the absence of this signal, even with high blood levels of both glucose and insulin, the liver begins to break down glycogen to be released as glucose into the blood, further increasing glucose and driving up insulin.

With fats, there's a different problem. Remember, when insulin comes to a healthy liver, the liver readily takes excess glucose and converts it to fat. Some of this fat will be stored in the liver, and some will be passed into the blood.[12] With the typical hyperinsulinemia that accompanies insulin resistance, this process is happening more often than normal. In other words, the excess insulin signals to the liver to create excess fat. This scenario creates two potentially dangerous problems, hyperlipidemia and fatty liver disease.

Hyperlipidemia

We discussed the role of insulin resistance in causing *dys*lipidemia earlier (see page 17)—insulin unfavorably changes cholesterol in the blood. *Hyper*lipidemia, on the other hand, means the blood has too much fat in general, often carried on lipoproteins (LDL cholesterol and its precursor VLDL cholesterol).

When the liver produces fat from any source, it commonly produces a saturated fat called palmitic acid. This isn't benign—increased saturated fat in the blood is potentially pathological, increasing inflammation and cardiovascular complications, and exacerbating insulin resistance. And importantly, this can happen even when a person eats absolutely no fat. (Saturated fat in the blood is not analogous to saturated fat in the diet, which we'll revisit.)

Nonalcoholic Fatty Liver Disease

Instead of secreting fat into the blood, the liver can store it. If the liver stores too much fat, it will start to lose functionality and may develop more serious complications. For the liver, "too much" fat is defined as 5% to 10% of its total weight consisting of fat.

Historically, developing a fatty liver was seen almost exclusively with excess alcohol consumption. No other tissue can metabolize alcohol, and over time drinking too much does lead to fat buildup in your liver cells, known as alcoholic fatty liver disease. However, you can get fatty liver disease even if you don't drink. And in recent decades, we've seen a shift; roughly one in three people in the United States has nonalcoholic fatty liver disease (NAFLD).[13] That number increases every year and is likely more prevalent than we think, considering that the disease is clinically silent in its early stages. This is utterly remarkable: A disease that was practically unheard of 30 years ago is now the most common liver disorder in Western countries.[14] It has much to do with insulin resistance.

FRUCTOSE: SICKENINGLY SWEET FOR THE LIVER

Fructose is similar to alcohol, but without the hangover. What the two have in common is where they're "handled"; both are metabolized by the liver. Unfortunately, the liver has very limited options for metabolizing fructose and alcohol; much of what isn't used for energy production is converted to fat. Indeed, just as alcohol causes alcoholic fatty liver disease, high fructose consumption is a potent contributor to NAFLD.[15] Fructose is so good at making the liver fat, that just one week of eating high-fructose foods is enough to make the liver observably fatter.

A phenomenal study published in 2009 explored the effect of fructose versus glucose on visceral fat.[16] The subjects received drinks containing either fructose or glucose. Unsurprisingly, the subjects all gained fat. However, the interesting detail was where the fat accumulated. While the glucose drinkers developed more subcutaneous fat, the fructose drinkers—you guessed it—developed more visceral fat. Tragically, we consume several times more fructose now than we did a generation ago.[17] Other than sugar (which is half fructose), the culprit is largely our love of fruit juice. Many of us consider it a healthy drink, but all fruit juice is a potent source of pure fructose. (Unfortunately, our misunderstanding is a significant part of why NAFLD is on the rise in *children* as well as adults.[18]) Hopefully this prompts you to think twice before drinking that cup of apple juice, let alone giving it to your kids![19] This is not, however, a call to avoid fruit. Because of its fiber content and relatively lower fructose, whole fruit is very different from fruit juice—in fact, eating whole fruit is better for improving diabetes risk than drinking juice from the same fruit. So eat your fruit, don't drink it.

THE MICROBREWERY IN YOUR BELLY

Imagine a situation where you drink no alcohol, yet you develop actual alcoholic fatty liver disease. This is just what happened with a man in China, where scientists stumbled onto the realization that their sober-minded subject wasn't so sober; he had chronically elevated blood alcohol despite not drinking any.[20] Remarkably, the man had a high level of a certain intestinal bacterium (*Klebsiella pneumoniae*) that ferments glucose to produce high levels of alcohol, which contributed to his developing fatty liver disease. And he's not alone—in this study, they found that up to 60% of the people studied with fatty liver disease had these same bacteria.

Being insulin resistant is the strongest known predictor of developing NAFLD, increasing the risk of having it by 15 times compared with an insulin-sensitive person. Critically, while almost all obese individuals have NAFLD, even lean people, if insulin resistant, have a substantially greater likelihood of developing the condition.[21] In fact, if a lean person is diagnosed with NAFLD, it is an almost certain sign the person has insulin resistance and will likely develop type 2 diabetes.

Fatty liver was once considered to be nothing more than a benign side effect of other diseases, but recent studies refute this idea. NAFLD is a gateway to more serious and potentially life-threatening liver disorders, all of which are associated with insulin resistance.[22] Once a person develops NAFLD, the liver can later become inflamed, which, if chronic, can lead to scarring of the liver, known as hepatic fibrosis. One-half of all people with NAFLD will develop fibrosis.[23] After this, one-fifth of people with NAFLD will develop cirrhosis, and then potential liver failure, requiring liver transplant for survival. In some, they may avoid liver failure but develop liver cancer[24]—not a good trade-off.

HEPATITIS C

The liver disorders we've covered are problems that develop over time as a result of insulin resistance. However, there are several known viral causes of liver infection that have nothing to do with insulin resistance: hepatitis viruses. While insulin resistance is certainly not relevant in the person *getting* the disease, there is limited evidence that insulin resistance may make the infection worse. For instance, in patients with hepatitis C, those who have insulin resistance experience the worst degree of fibrosis.[25] Moreover, insulin resistance may mitigate the benefits of antiviral medications.[26]

Insulin and the Gallbladder

The gallbladder, located right beneath the liver, is the liver's sidekick; they work together to properly digest the fats we eat. The gallbladder's main job is to store bile, a fluid created by the liver. Bile is mostly water along with salts, bilirubin (a substance made up of old red blood cells), and fats. These substances all act together to emulsify fats in the intestines so that they can be absorbed into the body. By acting as a reservoir for bile, the gallbladder allows the body to digest fat more readily than if the liver were forced to produce the required quantity each time.

The most common disorder of the gallbladder occurs when the otherwise very watery mix of bile becomes too thick, resulting in the formation of stones.

Gallstones

Bile can become prone to forming stones in two ways: the liver may be producing too much cholesterol, or the gallbladder may not be contracting enough to push bile into the intestines. Insulin resistance affects both of these functions.

First, let's look at the situation with excess cholesterol. A gallstone can form if the bile becomes too enriched with either bilirubin or cholesterol. The liver is responsible for removing old red blood cells from the body, and bilirubin is a part of a degraded red blood cell—insulin resistance has nothing to do with this (so far as I know). However, insulin has a tremendous influence on the rate of cholesterol production in the liver. The cholesterol can either enter the blood or be moved into the bile and stored in the gallbladder. Thus, as the body becomes insulin resistant and insulin levels climb, the liver begins producing more cholesterol than normal, which can enrich the bile with too much cholesterol.

Multiple human studies have found that insulin resistance is one of the most significant risk factors for developing gallstones,[27] predominantly cholesterol stones, the most common type worldwide. There's even clearer evidence in animal studies that insulin and insulin resistance directly cause gallstone formation. One study in hamsters found that injecting the animals with insulin daily for one week was sufficient to increase cholesterol gallstone formation.[28] In a second study, scientists created genetically modified mice that were insulin resistant only in the liver. They fed their rodent subjects a diet of cholesterol-enriched chow. The liver-insulin-resistant animals, but not the normal mice, developed massive cholesterol stones.[29]

The gallbladder is normally able to reduce the chances of a stone by contracting to pump bile into the intestines. This ensures that bile components, such as cholesterol, have less time to coalesce and form a stone.

GALLSTONES: WHAT'S FAT GOT TO DO WITH IT?

Gallstones have a lot to do with dietary fat. After a stone forms in a person's gallbladder, they will very often feel sharp pain, which is the sensation of the gallbladder trying to eject bile into the intestines while the stone is blocking the duct.

However, dietary fat is one of the best ways to prevent a gallstone from forming. When a person eats fat, the gallbladder empties itself; increased dietary fat raises gallbladder motility (or how often it contracts), which helps prevent stone formation.

All of this is why people who adopt a low-fat, low-calorie diet for weight loss (quite common) have an increased risk of gallstone formation and, eventually, may need to have the gallbladder removed.[30]

Insulin slows gallbladder motility. In fact, the more insulin resistant a person is, the less the gallbladder contracts—and that's true even in people who haven't been diagnosed with insulin resistance.[31] Research has shown that even a four-hour infusion of insulin, creating an acute state of hyperinsulinemia, reduces gallbladder function.[32]

PREGNANCY AND GALLSTONES

Pregnancy increases the risk of developing gallstones or a thicker bile termed "sludge," which is an early warning for stone formation.[33] Interestingly, the sludge resolves itself to normal consistency once the pregnancy is over. Think back to chapter four. What else gets worse throughout pregnancy and gets better once the baby is born? Yep, insulin resistance. In fact, insulin resistance is the most predictive factor in developing bile sludge and may be the primary cause of pregnancy-related gallstone formation.[34]

The liver is essential for regulating numerous nutrient processes (such as controlling blood glucose) and for removing certain toxins from the blood. However, when it comes to cleaning the blood, the liver doesn't work alone—the kidneys carry much of the "filtering" load, and, of course, they require normal insulin function to work properly.

Kidney Health

While the kidneys are not part of our GI tract, they occupy similar space in the body and share a similar role as the liver, removing toxins and metabolites from the blood and eliminating them via the urine. Beyond acting as a filter, the kidneys are involved in a remarkable number of bodily processes. They help regulate our blood volume, bone health, pH balance, and more. In short, when the kidneys don't work well, the body doesn't work well.

Kidney Stones

The kidneys have the dubious honor of being involved in what many consider to be the most painful problem one can suffer: the passing of a kidney stone. (In fact, ask a female friend who's gone through childbirth and passing a stone—I bet she tells you the stone was worse.)

Before the stone makes its excruciating pilgrimage from the kidney to the toilet, it has to be created in the kidney, a process known as urolithiasis. And this is where insulin resistance becomes a factor, because it leads to two subtle physiological changes that create ideal conditions for kidney stone formation.

First, high blood insulin increases the amount of blood calcium. Too much calcium can cause various problems, including affecting the heart; calcium also forms the most common type of kidney stone. Because high blood calcium is pathogenic, the kidneys are constantly filtering some and eliminating this excess in small amounts via the urine. Naturally, as calcium levels in the blood climb, the kidneys filter more calcium than normal. Eventually, a point is reached where freshly produced urine becomes supersaturated with calcium. At this point, the calcium starts to form crystals in the kidneys that become stones.

The specific way that too much insulin leads to too much calcium is interesting. Insulin increases our levels of parathyroid hormone[35] (and parathyroid hormone, in turn, can cause insulin resistance[36]). One of this hormone's main functions is to increase blood calcium by raising the amount of calcium we absorb from food in our intestines and by increasing calcium resorption from our bones.

The second link between insulin resistance and kidney stones is the effect it has on urine's measure of acidity or alkalinity, or pH. As a result of the kidneys' involvement in properly balancing bodily pH, the urine is more acidic than the rest of the body. We only have a vague idea of how insulin resistance is connected to changes in urinary pH. It's likely because kidneys in an insulin-resistant state are less able to produce molecules that counteract the acid in urine. As the urine pH changes to become more alkaline, the urine can dissolve less and less of the various molecules (calcium, urate, and so on); as a result, stones begin to form.

Kidney Failure

Kidney failure is a lethal loss of most functions, including filtering ability. Type 2 diabetes is the most common cause—so when we remember that type 2 diabetes is insulin resistance, it's only mildly surprising that insulin resistance increases the risk of kidney failure by 50%.[37] And the worse the insulin resistance, the higher the risk; the most insulin-resistant people have a four-times greater risk of developing kidney failure than those with mild insulin resistance.[38] Importantly, this happens even when glucose levels are still normal!

Exactly how insulin resistance leads to kidney failure is not yet understood. Although some lines of evidence point to kidney failure resulting from certain insulin resistance–induced complications, such as hypertension and hyperlipidemia, it may simply be a result of too much insulin. Insulin can increase the size and thickness of our kidneys' filtering apparatuses,[39] which makes it increasingly difficult for molecules to pass from the blood into the urine.

I really can't overstate how important this connection is. Compared with those possessing healthy kidneys, people with kidney failure are up to three times more likely to die, so we should want to diagnose any risk factor, like insulin resistance, as early as possible. If we're only relying on the usual suspect to determine risk (that is, high enough glucose to officially diagnose type 2 diabetes), it will likely be too late. Insulin levels, which can indicate insulin resistance years before glucose rises, must be measured.

Our digestive and urinary tracts are involved in fundamental processes necessary to survival: moving nutrients into and through the body and eliminating the waste from digesting and metabolizing these nutrients. When insulin resistance starts to change their function, the digestive and urinary processes become compromised, altering how we digest and absorb foods, and even changing how the kidneys filter waste and regulate the body's pH. Of course, once the food is digested and in the blood, it becomes material for the body to use or store—and depending on what we're eating, that can have meaningful metabolic consequences.

CHAPTER 8

The Metabolic
Syndrome and Obesity

FOR A ONCE-OBSCURE DISORDER, the metabolic syndrome seems to
be enjoying a boost in awareness. Medical literature is discussing it
more often, and it's being recognized even in lay media; one in three
US adults has it, and almost 90% of all adults have at least one feature
of it. The metabolic syndrome is actually a constellation of disorders.
The World Health Organization defines the metabolic syndrome by
two main criteria: first, the patient must have two of either high blood
pressure, dyslipidemia, central obesity, or low levels of protein in the
urine; and second, the patient must have insulin resistance.

That's right: insulin resistance + any two of those other problems
= metabolic syndrome. (In fact, insulin resistance is such a critical
component of the metabolic syndrome that it used to be known as
insulin resistance syndrome.)

Obesity, for its part, really requires no introduction—it's a villain
that everyone loves to hate (even if sometimes unfairly). Obesity has
become so prevalent that it's now more likely that someone will be
obese than starving.[1] In a way, obesity, an excess of fat on the body,
is a perfect representation of the metabolic consequences of insulin
resistance and hyperinsulinemia; insulin, among its many effects, is
a strong advocate of fat cell growth, blocking these cells from sharing their fat to be used by the body and instead telling them to grow.
However, as we will see, while obesity and insulin resistance often
walk hand in hand, their relationship is surprisingly complicated.

"NOT ENOUGH INSULIN"

A common expression with type 2 diabetes is that "the patient doesn't have enough insulin." This unfortunate expression is wildly misleading. While some people with type 2 diabetes may indeed have dangerously low insulin levels because of dysfunctional beta cells in the pancreas, the clear majority have perfectly functioning beta cells; they simply can't produce enough insulin to overcome their significant system-wide insulin resistance. Yet this "not enough" paradigm is what drives the treatment of type 2 diabetes with insulin, which, as you'll learn, is what makes the patient fatter, sicker, and ever more insulin resistant.

Giving a person with prediabetes and hyperinsulinemia, or one with type 2 diabetes, more insulin is like giving someone with hyperthyroidism, a disease of excess thyroid hormone, even more thyroid hormone. In other words, total nonsense. Rather than claiming there's "not enough insulin," a more accurate statement that would drive better approaches than insulin therapy would be, "Insulin is less effective—let's look at other treatments."

Obesity and Insulin Resistance: It's Complicated

Like every exciting relationship, the connection between insulin resistance and obesity is complicated—it's a chicken-and-egg question of which happens first.

That obesity and insulin resistance tend to occur together (an understatement) has been observed for roughly a century. There is no doubt that excess body fat is related to insulin resistance. Most overweight/obese individuals are insulin resistant (~70%), and because insulin resistance is so commonly associated with excess body fat, plenty of scientists have tried to find out why. But we only started looking at obesity and insulin resistance in a *causal* relationship within the last 30 years or so. Many of these researchers concluded that obesity drives insulin resistance. Indeed, this is the predominant perspective; the term "obesity-induced insulin resistance" comes up often in this area of research. An internet search for this term yields thousands of hits on search engines for biomedical research. Many of these studies report that insulin sensitivity improves because of weight loss.

But, as I suggested, it's not that simple. In looking at the data from these *same studies*, it is just as viable to conclude that weight loss occurred *because* of improved insulin sensitivity—not the other way around. And indeed, some studies do acknowledge a possibility that insulin resistance may come before the subjects' weight gain (or insulin sensitivity may precede their weight loss).[2] In one instance, scientists measured several variables in a group of children and then followed up almost 10 years later. Even if kids weighed the same or grew the same amount, those with the highest insulin levels were the most likely to gain the most weight. In fact, in a similar study, though their body weight was similar at the beginning, children with the highest insulin levels were 36 times more likely to become obese as adults.[3]

However, the data become murky when we look at adults, but one interesting study sheds some light. By following adults over several years, scientists in Boston found that when insulin was lower, body weight gain was slower; when insulin was higher, body weight gain was higher.[4] However, as adults gain ever more weight and weight gain reaches a limit, insulin loses its predictive power.[5] This limit for weight gain is known as the "personal fat threshold," and it represents a sort of cold war between our fat tissue and insulin resistance (we'll revisit and expand this in chapter eleven).

Although the evidence that high blood insulin precedes obesity, and thus could be causal, is robust, this perspective is not without debate. (For more on this perspective, I recommend reading Gary Taubes's *Good Calories, Bad Calories*, Dr. Jason Fung's *The Obesity Code*, Dr. David Ludwig's *Always Hungry?*, or Dr. Stephan Guyenet's *The Hungry Brain*). Another theory is far more popular and widely embraced among health professionals and the general public alike—and we've been stuck on this theory for decades.

Why Do We Get Fat?

The history of obesity research and treatment is as fascinating as it is unfortunate. It was once widely accepted that obesity was at least partly a hormone problem; in 1923, Dr. Wilhelm Falta, a prominent internist in Vienna, noted that "for fattening . . . is necessary [to have] an intact pancreas"[6] (I'll add that he meant "the hormones from the pancreas"). However, in the mid-1900s, there was a dramatic shift in thinking that settled on our current prevailing dogma—the "calories in, calories out" perspective that holds obesity is simply a result of ingesting more calories than are expended. In other words, the theory goes, if we eat more than we burn, we'll gain fat; we can only lose fat if we eat less than we burn.

This makes a certain amount of sense considering we define body fat as a biological caloric reservoir—a place to store calories for later use. Further, it fits our understanding of energy use and storage. If you throw less wood (fuel) on the fire, there's less to burn. Unfortunately, this theory ignores the complex processes in the body that regulate how it uses fuel; the body is a little more complicated than a campfire.

Ultimately, hormones determine what the body does with the fuel we eat and store—whether it is making more muscle, making bigger bones, making more fat, dissipating it as heat, and so on. There are thousands of known hormones, with more being discovered all the time. While most have nothing to do with how we use calories, many do, and no single signal promotes fat cells to grow as much as insulin does.

LEPTIN RESISTANCE

Leptin, from the Greek word for "thin" (*leptos*), was once considered the great solution to the obesity epidemic. For the *very* few people with an inability to produce leptin, it is. However, for the vast majority of people who struggle with their weight, it is not a solution.

In fact, most obese people have *elevated* leptin levels, not reduced. However, leptin is no longer as effective in obese people as it once was in regulating appetite and metabolic processes. One key process is leptin's inhibition of insulin; leptin is supposed to prevent insulin secretion, which will help keep a person thin.[7] However, with too much leptin for too long, the body becomes leptin resistant, and leptin is progressively less able to prevent insulin secretion,[8] all of which leads to fat gain.

Unfortunately, this is a vicious cycle. If leptin resistance stems from chronically elevated levels of leptin, what increases the leptin in the first place? Insulin, of course; insulin naturally stimulates leptin production from fat tissue, so too much insulin leads to too much leptin.

The starkest examples of how insulin drives body fat are the two typical types of diabetes mellitus. (Remember, type 1 is a disease of too little insulin, and type 2 is a disease of too much.)

In the case of a type 1 diabetes patient, unless they take their insulin injections, they can't get fat. Not even a bit. In fact, some people with type 1 diabetes are so terribly aware of this fact and so determined to stay thin, that they intentionally underdose insulin in order to avoid gaining fat regardless of the amount or type of food they consume[9]; this is an eating disorder called diabulimia. Type 1 diabetes often manifests in the second decade, when the person, as a teenager, is more mindful of body image than ever. Unfortunately, despite being as lean as he or she wants, the person experiences massive hyperglycemia—glucose levels can be up to 10 times higher than normal. While this book focuses on the negatives of too much insulin, too much glucose is certainly also problematic. Many people with chronic diabulimia endure kidney failure, blindness, and even limb amputation. Furthermore, independent of the glucose, too little or no insulin results in dangerous changes in blood pH, causing potentially lethal acidosis.

In contrast to the type 1 diabetes patients staying lean without insulin, those with type 2 diabetes who have been prescribed insulin to control blood glucose will gain weight.[10] The aim for these patients is finding the insulin regimen that results in the least amount of fat gain. Once type 2 diabetes patients start to notice weight gain, some may attempt to correct the problem by eating less. However, as the insulin injections are making their bodies ever more insulin resistant, they will need ever more insulin to control blood glucose, and even eating less won't be sufficient to prevent the insulin-induced fat gain.[11]

Bottom line: When it comes to body fat, the hormone insulin is the critical factor—if insulin is up, body fat goes up; if insulin is down, body fat goes down. Indeed, insulin is so good at increasing body fat that rising amounts of insulin increase body fat even when the number of calories consumed stays the same.[12] To make this point clear, if person A is eating a 2,500-calorie diet that keeps insulin low, person A will be leaner than person B, who is eating a 2,500-calorie diet that keeps insulin high. (We'll look at that diet in more detail in Part II.) Simply put, insulin directs nutrients toward being stored as fat.

Of course, as we'll see later, it is still true that obesity leads to insulin resistance. But it's important that we understand it works both ways. This alternative paradigm is more than semantics. It represents a fundamental shift in how we view the relationship between obesity and insulin resistance; it would alter how we view the origins of insulin resistance and give us a better understanding of how to fight it.

In fact, we've reached that point. Having positioned insulin resistance as the villain, it's time for the origin story; how did such a nice, normal process like insulin signaling go so wrong?

PART II

Causes
What Makes Us Insulin Resistant in the First Place?

CHAPTER 9

How Age and Genetics Influence Insulin

By now, we've seen that insulin resistance is at the root of many of the chronic diseases that are unfortunately becoming all too common. And so, the question becomes: How did we get here? What exactly makes a body become insulin resistant? And more importantly, can it be stopped?

Considering how common insulin resistance has become, researchers have devoted substantial attention to understanding how it develops. Some of these discoveries have been unexpected (such as the actual role of genetics—spoiler alert: it's not as important as you think), while others have been more of a rediscovery of lessons from the past (like the importance of a healthy lifestyle). Moreover, while some of these causes are unavoidable, others, thankfully, are well within our control. All are worth exploring.

Let's start the discussion on a depressing note—the things we can do nothing about! We all age, and, for better and worse, we all inherited the genes our parents gave us. My intention in this chapter is not to discourage; rather, I want to make you aware of the factors beyond your control so that (I hope!) you'll be that much more determined to make the changes you *can* control that really count.

Genetics

Ah, genetics—another reason to be frustrated with our parents.

There is no doubt that if your mom and dad are insulin resistant, you'll likely struggle with it, too. In a study of insulin resistance in early teenage children, children with at least one parent with insulin resistance were themselves more insulin resistant, with fasting insulin levels roughly 20% higher than levels in children who had no parents with insulin resistance.[1] Other studies have explored the role of familial genetics in a rather compelling way—by looking at identical twins. As you'd expect, individuals who are genetically the same, but who might be raised in different homes, have a very high likelihood of developing similar health problems, including insulin resistance.[2]

Importantly, genetic mutations that cause insulin resistance are very rare—these account for approximately 5% of all cases of type 2 diabetes (and even fewer cases of prediabetes/insulin resistance).[3] For the rest of us who have "garden variety" insulin resistance, which is the vast majority of cases, our genes are not as important as what we do with them—the old battle between genetics and environment, nature versus nurture. In other words, it's one thing to have genes that might increase our likelihood of developing insulin resistance, but it's another to put those genes into the wrong lifestyle. Our daily decisions matter at least as much as our genetics, as we will see.

Ethnicity

Interestingly, certain ethnicities, which can carry multiple specific genetic traits, tend to have an increased likelihood of becoming insulin resistant. One notable study compared the insulin sensitivity (among other things) of four prominent ethnicities in the United States— Hispanic, Asian, African, and "Caucasian" (which might more accurately be defined as "Northern European").[4] Despite having roughly similar body weights and waist-to-hip ratios among all the groups, the most insulin-resistant group was Hispanic Americans. The next most insulin resistant group was the Asian American group, which is interesting because they were also the group with the lowest (though not statistically significant) body weight and waist-to-hip ratio. African Americans were the third most insulin-resistant group, with Caucasians being the least insulin resistant. In most groups, obesity and waist-to-hip ratio are very highly correlated with insulin resistance, and this is what we'd expect. However, the Asian group seems not to play by the same rules. This group had the lowest waist-to-hip ratios and BMIs, and yet were surprisingly more likely to be insulin resistant.

(We'll learn more about waist-to-hip ratio in chapter eleven; see the box on page 105.)

But this study did not include other ethnicities that warrant mention, namely the Pima Indians, an indigenous American people who generally live in southern Arizona. This group has the highest prevalence of insulin resistance of any group in America. Insulin resistance is such a problem among this group that children as young as four years old have been diagnosed with type 2 diabetes.[5]

The remarkably common observation of insulin resistance among the Pima and other Native Americans led in the 1980s to a now-famous theory known as the "thrifty genotype."[6] Genotype is the scientific term that simply means "the genes that we have." The theory was posited in an effort to understand why some people, like Native Americans, have such a pronounced collective risk of insulin resistance and type 2 diabetes. At its foundation, the theory is built on the idea that because of repeated cycles of "feast or famine" periods—times when food was sparse punctuated by brief moments of plenty—people developed the ability to efficiently store energy from food as fat. This would allow a person to have energy to use during times when food is insufficient. And the high insulin levels that go along with insulin resistance signal the body to store energy.

However, this theory is by no means proven and has been repeatedly challenged. As a counterpoint, consider people who have high rates of insulin resistance yet have likely never experienced feast–famine cycles because of their location. A perfect example of this is Pacific Islanders, some of whom have the absolute highest rates of insulin resistance in the world, despite living in a climate and location that provides ample edible vegetation and fish year round.[7] This phenomenon among Pacific Islanders led researchers to wonder if insulin resistance among certain populations has less to do with their genes being prone to storing fat than it does to their becoming adapted to certain foods.

This alternative theory is built on the very real facts that insulin resistance is becoming increasingly common among people who have been exposed more recently to a Western diet. Insulin resistance is relatively lower among people of European descent, though it has certainly increased over time. Thus, the theory would suggest that while those of European descent have had more time to adapt to foods that can raise insulin and lead to diabetes, populations that were exposed to these foods more recently (within the last 100 years or so) are suffering the consequences more dramatically. A comparison within the various populations reveals that people who have emigrated and adopted a Western diet invariably have higher rates of insulin resistance than their counterparts in their countries of origin following a more traditional lifestyle and diet.

Thankfully, as complicated as the genetics–insulin resistance web may be, understanding how age impacts insulin resistance is a little clearer, albeit similarly frustrating. As futile as it is to try to stay young, understanding how age and insulin resistance connect can give us an edge in combating insulin resistance as we grow older.

Age

Growing old isn't for the faint of heart. As we saw in chapter six, aging is a very complicated process that encompasses countless subtle and not-so-subtle physical and mental changes, including thinning or graying hair, weaker and wrinkled skin, and a certain propensity to misplace one's keys . . .

Among these several unpleasant changes are certain metabolic alterations, including changes in insulin sensitivity; as we've seen, it may even cause some aging symptoms. As with weight gain, this works both ways; the older we get, the more insulin resistant we generally become.[8] A number of aging processes and common conditions can contribute to the development of insulin resistance, including age-related muscle loss (sarcopenia) and the hormonal changes that occur with age. However, unlike so many changes, insulin resistance may not be a required part of aging—it's a process we can fight.

Hormone Changes in Aging Women: How Menopause Increases Insulin Resistance

Menopause is the unavoidable constellation of changes that marks the end of a woman's reproductive years. Menopause also serves as a fascinating example of how intimately our metabolic and reproductive processes are linked—when one is altered, the other usually follows.

Several physical changes accompany the altered hormone production in the ovaries, which is predominantly marked by a loss of estrogens. A small family of hormones, estrogens not only help the female body maintain normal function in a variety of areas, such as reproduction, but they also potently affect metabolic function.

HOT FLASHES: AS IF THE SWEATING WEREN'T BAD ENOUGH

In a study of more than 3,000 middle-aged women, study subjects experiencing hot flashes were significantly more likely to experience insulin resistance.[9] Importantly, the hot flash–insulin resistance connection persisted independent of estrogen levels and body mass.

In both men and women, estrogen helps maintain insulin sensitivity. We can see strong evidence of this in people whose bodies are *incapable* of producing estrogens due to a deficiency in aromatase, the enzyme that converts androgens to estrogens. The inability to produce estrogens, in addition to other effects, causes insulin resistance to develop.[10]

Of course, estrogen changes in menopause aren't quite this dramatic. Nevertheless, the reduction in estrogen is sufficient to make a woman more insulin resistant than she would otherwise be,[11] and artificially maintaining high estrogens with hormone therapy partially helps maintain insulin sensitivity through menopause[12] (though as we'll explore, it's certainly not the only method).

Hormone Changes in Aging Men: How Testosterone Changes Insulin Resistance

Some consider the decrease in testosterone that occurs in aging men to be a type of male menopause. Analogous to the woman whose body is changing due to the reduction in estrogens, the man's body changes due to the loss of testosterone. Among these changes is increased insulin resistance.[13] By treating the man with testosterone, one is able to mitigate these negative effects and improve insulin sensitivity.[14]

However, more and more men lately are being diagnosed as having "low testosterone." In addition to becoming incredibly common, it's showing up in much younger men—they're not "old" by standard definitions of male aging (I have to believe that over 40 isn't *that* old . . .). Importantly, this is a recent phenomenon, largely a consequence of our altered diet and lifestyle. (Later, we'll explore the role of lifestyle in creating this state of "low testosterone," which has far less to do with aging per se and far more to do with how the man is aging.)

Like the weather, it's pointless to fight our genetics or age, though that doesn't mean we can't be prepared with a plan (coming up). As you've learned, at least some of the effect of aging on insulin resistance is through changes in sex hormones. As powerful as these age-related changes in sex hormones are, insulin—a hormone itself—also has a complicated relationship with several other hormones. Get ready for a peek into these torrid affairs.

CHAPTER 10

How Hormones Cause Insulin Resistance

HERE'S A BASIC PHYSIOLOGY LESSON: hormones affect hormones. There are certainly nonhormonal influences, such as stress or sleep deprivation, but once bodily levels of one hormone start to change, it starts pulling other hormones out onto the dance floor. Because insulin is so central in controlling metabolic function in the body, it's no surprise that insulin is a popular dance partner—everyone seems to want insulin's attention. Including insulin itself.

Too Much Insulin Causes Insulin Resistance

Of the various factors that can cause insulin resistance, insulin itself is the most relevant. Perhaps this won't surprise you by now, but, to state the obvious: too much insulin causes insulin resistance. To be precise about it, for every 1-microunit (μU) increase in fasting blood insulin (a pretty small change), a person can experience an approximately 20% increase in insulin resistance.[1] This might seem like a strange cause and effect, but it represents a fundamental feature of how the body works: when a process is excessively activated, the body will often dampen its response to the excess stimulus in order to reduce the activation. (This is similar to how bacteria become resistant to antibiotics or how, over time, a caffeine addict will need more caffeine than she used to.) If a cell, such as those of the muscle or liver, is inundated with insulin, it can do nothing to directly reduce the insulin the pancreas is producing. But it can alter *itself* to ensure that insulin has a smaller effect; thus, it becomes resistant to insulin. As this occurs in countless cells in tissues throughout the body, the body as a whole becomes insulin resistant.

One of the most convincing examples of this is when someone suffers from an insulin-producing tumor of the pancreas. In this instance, known as an insulinoma, the beta cells are constantly pumping insulin into the blood and ignoring signals (like reduced blood glucose) that would normally turn insulin down. The patients with the highest degree of insulin production from the insulinoma become highly insulin resistant, whereas the patients with the lower insulin levels become mildly insulin resistant. But, in the end, they always develop insulin resistance.[2]

Perhaps the rarest case of insulin driving insulin resistance is hypothalamic obesity, a terrible condition in which a person has accidental damage to a distinct region of the brain known as the ventromedial hypothalamus (VMH). This brain region has direct control over the pancreas via the vagus nerve. In particular, when the VMH is damaged, be it through tumors, brain surgery, or trauma, the VMH loses its control over the vagus nerve, which begins stimulating constant insulin secretion. In addition to substantial weight gain, this artificial increase in insulin leads to profound insulin resistance.[3]

In a more academic setting, scientists induced hyperinsulinemia by infusing healthy insulin-sensitive men with insulin for a prolonged period.[4] Even though the insulin dose was at a level we normally reach in a day, by keeping a steady infusion, the men became insulin resistant after just a few hours. On its face, this scenario might seem somewhat unrealistic; after all, nobody normally sits in a chair while receiving an insulin infusion. But it's a lab-created reflection of a condition that might seem familiar in another context—say, if a person were sitting in a chair and snacking often on insulin-spiking foods.

What's more, as we have seen, the common (but misguided) method of treating type 2 diabetes is to give the patient insulin injections. Having people with type 2 diabetes take insulin creates an artificially high state of insulin (higher than the pancreas alone could ever produce), which is then sufficient to bring blood glucose under control—for a time. However, because insulin causes insulin resistance, the insulin injections are increasing the person's insulin resistance, which over time creates a demand for higher insulin doses, creating a vicious cycle.[5] Interestingly, this can even happen in type 1 diabetes, which *must* be treated with insulin. But if these patients eat a diet that forces them to inject high amounts of insulin to control their glucose levels, they'll become insulin resistant, a condition sometimes referred to as "double diabetes."[6]

ARE YOUR BETA CELLS REALLY GONE?

Many people with type 2 diabetes have been led to understand that the reason their glucose levels have climbed to a critical level is that their pancreas isn't making enough insulin. This is partly true, but also misleading. The fact is that most people with type 2 diabetes, and certainly those with prediabetes (that is, those with insulin resistance), have high levels of insulin.[7] Thus, the problem isn't that the beta cells are dying, but rather they simply can't produce enough insulin to keep blood glucose levels under control.

Extracted beta cells that are cultivated in isolated laboratory conditions provide an interesting model to help us understand what happens to beta cells with insulin resistance. When you expose beta cells to high levels of glucose for a long time, they start to shut down. How do you restore them? Yep, it's as simple as lowering the glucose.[8]

Of course, we're more complicated as an organism than just our beta cells. However, the same thing appears to happen when we look at people. A study in the UK found that type 2 diabetes patients with reduced beta cell function had a "normalization of . . . beta cell function" simply by restricting carbohydrates (and therefore glucose) for eight weeks.[9] Another study even identified the specific proteins that allow the beta cells in an insulin-resistant person (that is, one with type 2 diabetes) to recover.[10]

However, the ability of the beta cells to "rebound" may not be universal. In another study of type 2 diabetes patients on a carbohydrate-restricted diet, roughly half experienced the expected recovery, while the other half still required medication—albeit less than before.[11]

What all these improvements have in common is that the beta cells of the pancreas are given a rest. By controlling carbohydrates, the beta cells are allowed to enjoy a reduced-glucose condition that doesn't force them to work so hard.[12]

> If you have type 2 diabetes and use insulin, it's possible (though unlikely) your beta cells are gone for good or they may be waiting for that well-earned rest before coming back to work. You won't know until you try.

In the end, regardless of where the increase in insulin starts, insulin resistance is the result. The evidence is clear that too much insulin drives insulin resistance at several parts of the body, including muscle and fat tissue, which we'll explore more in chapter eleven.

Critically, the high insulin doesn't only arise from an overt medical problem, but most often stems simply from lifestyle. Unfortunately, as we'll see in later chapters, our current lifestyle is a perfect storm of hyperinsulinemia.

But we're getting ahead of ourselves—other hormones can cause insulin resistance. Remember, insulin isn't just dancing alone; other hormones are all lined up for the belle of the hormone ball. Let's see what tune they dance to!

The Stress Hormones: Epinephrine and Cortisol

The stress response involves an interesting mix of neural and endocrine (hormone) events. We'll look at two in particular: epinephrine and cortisol, both of which come from the adrenal glands.

In the earliest stages of stress, epinephrine increases heart rate and blood pressure. But too much epinephrine for too long is capable of causing insulin resistance. In one study from Yale University, healthy men underwent several assessments to measure insulin sensitivity with or without an infusion of epinephrine. After just two hours of epinephrine infusion, insulin sensitivity dropped by over 40%.[13]

While stress causes multiple hormones to be released into the blood, cortisol is considered the prototypical stress hormone, and many of the consequences of long-term stress are a result of its actions on the body. Cortisol wants us to have enough energy to get us through what we perceive to be a stressful situation. To get us that energy, cortisol is determined to raise our blood glucose—and so the hormone will tell the liver to make glucose out of anything it can get, including amino acids (from muscle protein) and glycerol (from fats).

While cortisol is trying to increase blood glucose, insulin is trying to reduce blood glucose. These two hormones are counter-regulatory: they act against each other. But in this fight, cortisol wins; cortisol makes the body remarkably insulin resistant, which is associated with a steady increase in blood insulin over time.[14] One of the more dramatic examples of this scenario is Cushing's syndrome—a family of disorders that results from the adrenal glands producing too much cortisol. As you would expect, individuals who develop Cushing's syndrome, whether as a result of a hormone issue or another abnormality, go from being perfectly insulin sensitive to highly insulin resistant after the cortisol starts to climb.[15]

CORTISOL AND BAD FAT

We generally store fat in two areas on our bodies: beneath our skin, called subcutaneous fat, and around our internal organs, called visceral fat. Cortisol is known to cause insulin resistance directly, but it also selectively drives visceral fat to grow more than subcutaneous fat, creating an unhealthy metabolic state.[16]

That the two main stress hormones cause insulin resistance makes a certain sense. Imagine if you were forced to flee a dangerous situation; you would benefit from the effects of cortisol and epinephrine, which would instantly cooperate to increase blood glucose and fats, feeding your muscles a readily used fuel to help you escape. If insulin were high in that condition, that glucose would be pushed into tissues that don't need it, particularly fat tissue. But by making the body insulin resistant, these stress hormones ensure that the tissue that needs fuel, such as the muscle, can get it (which it does through insulin-independent mechanisms while contracting). Unfortunately, the effects of cortisol are the same regardless of the situation we perceive as stressful—whether it's something as urgent as running away from a predator or as seemingly benign as arguing with a loved one or even staying up late studying. Thus, while a stress response in a genuinely dangerous situation serves a purpose to fuel the body's actions, in these instances of modern stress, the metabolic consequences of a stress response simply make things worse—all this available fat and glucose with nowhere to go.

But a hormone doesn't have to be related to stress for it to fight insulin's actions. In fact, sometimes a hormone helps insulin work better—a hormone insulin actually wants to dance with.

Thyroid Hormone

Thyroid hormone does multiple things throughout the body; in fact, all cells respond to it. Thyroid hormone alters cardiovascular function, regulates the nervous system, and is essential for healthy reproduction. But most of us think of the thyroid's actions only in the context of metabolic function, as a cause of weight gain. While it's true that thyroid hormone acts as a sort of metabolic choke valve—it can increase or decrease metabolic rate by altering the rate at which a cell is working—this having a meaningful influence on the modern obesity epidemic is very unlikely, as thyroid levels in obese individuals are often normal. Less well known are the thyroid's effects on insulin sensitivity.

THYROID RESISTANCE

On average, the more fat you have, the more active the thyroid gland.[17] This is a type of "thyroid resistance," where the body is less responsive to the regulation of thyroid hormone. Interestingly, losing weight tends to reduce thyroid levels, suggesting that the body is more sensitive and thyroid hormone is more effective.[18]

Having too little thyroid hormone (hypothyroidism) is associated with reduced insulin sensitivity.[19] With less thyroid hormone production, the average cell will have fewer insulin receptors, which means insulin has a smaller effect. As a result, the pancreas will make more insulin in an effort to elicit a desired action, such as controlling blood glucose. Of course, with fewer receptors, the increased amount of insulin won't solve the problem—there are simply too few places for insulin to act. This feature of hypothyroidism is important; as we saw in Part I, insulin resistance is connected to multiple chronic and potentially lethal diseases. Because hypothyroidism is a cause of insulin resistance, understanding insulin resistance can help mitigate some of the complications typically associated with hypothyroidism.

Importantly, hypothyroidism changes the way fat cells respond to insulin in a particular manner. With hypothyroidism, fat cells take up less glucose in response to insulin, but insulin is still able to block fat breakdown in the fat cell, preventing the cell from shrinking. So, as blood insulin levels increase with hypothyroidism, it also very effectively prevents fat loss.

On the other end of the spectrum, too much thyroid hormone, or hyperthyroidism, results in roughly 70% more insulin receptors on fat cells.[20] This means that each fat cell may be 70% more responsive to the fat-cell-growing effects of insulin, which potentially improves insulin sensitivity (as we'll discuss later, fat cells that can keep getting fat are a good thing for insulin resistance). The critical connection between insulin and obesity is not a key topic in this book, though it is essential in understanding the true cause of obesity, which is more nuanced than simple caloric balance.

Some hormones play nicely with insulin and some don't, but this reflects the nuanced and delicate interaction of hormones within the body. While stress hormones tend to oppose insulin's actions and drive insulin resistance, thyroid hormone has a more favorable, albeit complicated relationship. Throughout this hormone discussion, we've been mentioning fat cells and how hormones regulate their function; well, it's time to stop skirting around the fat cell and dive right in. Hold your breath!

CHAPTER 11

Obesity and Insulin Resistance, Revisited

N OW, I KNOW WHAT YOU'RE THINKING: "Didn't we already talk about obesity? How can obesity be a *cause* of insulin resistance if it's a *consequence* of insulin resistance?"

My answer, again: it's complicated! Insulin resistance and obesity have a very strong connection, but which comes first is a matter of some debate. There is evidence to support both perspectives. In chapter nine, we explored how high insulin levels lead to the accumulation of body fat. Now, it's time to review the evidence on the other (more widely accepted) side of the story: how obesity causes insulin resistance.

Location Matters

As with real estate, so it is with body fat—it's all about location. We appreciate more than ever that excess body fat is largely relevant only if we store our fat in the wrong place. Where we store our fat is determined largely by our sex, partly by our genetics ("thanks, Mom and Dad"), and partly by diet.

Typically, we consider two predominant "patterns" of fat storage, referred to as fat deposition, although there are always exceptions (and some may have the misfortune of having both). A key difference between these two types of fat storage patterns is specific placement of the fat.

The "gynecoid" fat pattern is the result of fat stored beneath the skin, referred to as "subcutaneous fat." This pattern is typified by fat accumulating on the hips and thighs, with less fat on the upper body and trunk. Think of the pear shape typically seen with women due to the actions of estrogen.

In contrast, the "android" pattern may have both subcutaneous and visceral fat—meaning fat inside the trunk of the body, surrounding the visceral organs (liver, kidneys, intestines, and heart). This is the typical male fat storage pattern, analogous to the apple body shape. Someone with the android pattern stores most of their body fat right around the middle of the body—the "inner tube."

IF IT JIGGLES, IT'S GOOD

The best way to know which is your predominant fat pattern is simply to grab it. Yep. Grab it. (Only on yourself, please!)

If you can grab some fat and shake it, it's subcutaneous fat (= better). If you can't easily grab it or your belly is hard but big, it's likely you have more visceral fat (= worse).

So don't be so quick to curse jiggly body fat. We might not like how it looks or bulges, but it's better than the alternative.

We have long known that women have a better chance of living longer, healthier lives than men; this is partly due to the inherent differences in the impact these fat deposits have on insulin resistance and the subsequent risk of various chronic diseases. Ultimately, what is so important about these two fat patterns is the likelihood of having excess visceral fat. Study after study has shown that storing fat inside the core of the body is harmful, and we now know that there are differences in how fat behaves when it's stored in the viscera. And because men have a greater likelihood of storing fat there, this, in turn, is likely why men suffer more health problems with excess body fat than women do. A series of rodent experiments have established this. When visceral fat from an obese animal is transplanted into a lean animal, the recipient animal becomes insulin resistant immediately.[1] In contrast, when subcutaneous fat is transplanted into the lean animal, it remains insulin sensitive.[2]

Interestingly, these same rules apply to a seemingly lean person. That's right—even some people who look lean may be insulin resistant because of having more visceral fat. But wait: even lean individuals with insulin resistance are likely fatter than their lean insulin-sensitive counterparts. It's really a matter of whether you see the fat or not. And this is relevant because it emphasizes the most important aspect of obesity and insulin resistance; namely, where you're fat.

WAIST-TO-HIP RATIO

Want to know how you're doing? Another easy method to determine your fat pattern is to compare your girth around the largest part of your belly (near the navel; this is the waist measurement) with the largest part around your hips/buttocks (this is the hip measurement). Divide the waist number by the hip number. For example, if my waist is 30 inches and my hips are 40 inches, my waist-to-hip ratio is 0.75.

For men, this number is ideally below 0.9. For women, this number should be below 0.8.

Ultimately, the story still isn't over—it's not enough to know that excess body fat increases the risk of developing insulin resistance. We need to know how the fat leads to insulin resistance. Excess body fat, especially visceral fat, increases two pathological conditions—it increases inflammation and causes oxidative stress (covered in the next two chapters).

Fat Cell Size Matters

Did you know that your fat cells may be able to hold only so much fat? Like an overflowing cup, when your fat cells are "full," the excess fat begins spilling over into the blood and potentially getting stored in other tissues. The precise process is being actively studied, but the most consistent results suggest that it's because the fat cells simply become insulin resistant.

Insulin sends a powerful signal to the fat cell to store fat, which means to both pull fat in directly from the blood and to make new fat from glucose. However, insulin also slams the "exit" doors closed to prevent any fat from leaving, inhibiting the fat-shrinking process known as "lipolysis."

There is a fascinating and even obvious (as long as you have a microscope!) difference between fat cells that are insulin sensitive and continuing to store fat and those that are insulin resistant and "leaking" fat—it's all about size. As we gain fat, our fat tissue can grow in two ways: either via an increased number of fat cells (yet the fat cells themselves remain small; this is called "hyperplasia") or a growth in cell size (yet the number of fat cells remains lower; this is called "hypertrophy"). Larger fat cells have relatively fewer insulin receptors, for their size, than smaller fat cells.[3] Because of this, larger fat cells may not receive sufficient insulin stimulus, and as a result, the larger fat cells experience a degree of fat breakdown despite the presence of insulin attempting to block the process.

This series of events is evidence of a personal fat threshold—a limit to the size of the fat cells (and fat mass, by extension).[4] When a fat cell reaches its maximum dimensions through hypertrophy (which is several times that of the normal fat cell), it attempts to limit further growth; an excellent way to do this is to become resistant to insulin's growth signal. However, if fat cells can multiply via hyperplasia, they never reach this limit and maintain sensitivity. An interesting scenario plays out when we explore this idea in more detail. Let's imagine two people: one with fat cell hypertrophy and another with fat cell hyperplasia. The first fellow, whose fat is growing via hypertrophy, will stop gaining weight as the enlarged fat cells become insulin resistant and refuse to grow any further; this person could be only moderately overweight (by conventional standards), yet be very insulin resistant. In contrast, the second fellow, whose fat cells are multiplying, will continue to gain weight, and have a greater potential be very overweight, yet likely maintain a high degree of insulin sensitivity.

We can actually "hijack" this process with modern medicine. In a fascinating example of the power of fat cell size in determining insulin sensitivity and metabolic health, insulin-resistant patients are sometimes prescribed a type of medication ("thiazolidinediones"; discussed more in chapter sixteen) that actually forces the fat cells toward hyperplasia. Following this, an interesting scenario ensues: patients start gaining weight but become more insulin sensitive.[5] The drugs help fat cells continue to proliferate and store fat, which helps with insulin control, but, unfortunately, hurts weight control.

Importantly, the insulin-resistant fat cell that's grown beyond its borders not only leaks fat, but because it's "too big," it also becomes inflamed, dumping inflammatory proteins into the blood.[6] In the end, this means that the body is receiving this toxic mix of too much fat and too much inflammation, both of which drive insulin resistance.

THE "FAT FORMULA"

You might be able to determine your own fat tissue's insulin resistance with numbers from a blood test. If you can, next time you have a blood test, ask your healthcare provider to measure your insulin levels (in microunits per milliliter or µU/mL) and your free fatty acids (in millimoles per liter or mmol/L); with these numbers, you have what you need. Normally, insulin prevents fat cells from shedding their fat, which comes in the form of free fatty acids. Of course, if the fat cells are becoming insulin resistant, insulin may be high, and because it's not working too well, free fatty acids would be high. A recent publication found that a "fat formula" score of 9.3 (insulin × free fatty acids) was the optimal cutoff[7]; if your score is lower than 9.3, you can take some comfort that your fat cells are doing OK.

But why might fat cells grow in size and not number? What makes them "turn bad"? From what we've learned, there are a couple of known causes. Paradoxically, two distinct fat products can hurt the fat cell's ability to store fat in a healthy way, forcing fat cells to stop growing in number and start growing in size.

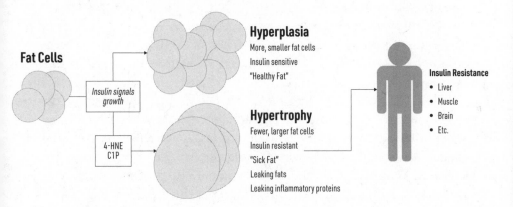

Fat Cells

Insulin signals growth

4-HNE
C1P

Hyperplasia
More, smaller fat cells
Insulin sensitive
"Healthy Fat"

Hypertrophy
Fewer, larger fat cells
Insulin resistant
"Sick Fat"
Leaking fats
Leaking inflammatory proteins

Insulin Resistance
• Liver
• Muscle
• Brain
• Etc.

Before we look at what these fat molecules do, a brief biochemistry lesson may be helpful. A fatty acid is the technical term for an individual fat molecule. Each molecule consists of a row of carbon atoms with hydrogen atoms linked to them. The number of hydrogens can differ between molecules, which is a sign of whether the fatty acid is saturated (having the maximum number of hydrogens) or unsaturated (having less than the maximum).

The first, and likely the worst, fat molecule that makes fat cells hypertrophy is called 4-hydroxynonenal (4-HNE).[8] 4-HNE is the little monster that is born from the unholy union of a polyunsaturated fat (such as an omega-6 fat) and reactive oxygen molecules (or oxidative stress). Because of the unique structure of the fat—that is, all the unsaturated bonds—and the positioning of those bonds, omega-6 fats are very, very readily oxidized.[9] Importantly, linoleic acid, the omega-6 fat of interest, is a massive part of our diet. It is the single most common fat consumed in the standard Western diet; it's essentially the main fat in all processed and packaged foods. And, not surprisingly, it has become a significant part of the fat we store in our fat cells, constituting roughly one quarter of it[10] (it's increased almost 150% in the last 50 years). With this in mind, it's easy to see the sequence: reactive oxygen molecules bump into the highly prevalent stored linoleic acid, creating 4-HNE, which accumulates and disrupts the fat cell's ability to proliferate, forcing it to grow in size rather than number.

The second fat character that disrupts fat cell growth, forcing hypertrophy, is called ceramide 1-phosphate (C1P). Whereas 4-HNE is a consequence of oxidative stress, C1P can be considered more a consequence of inflammation. Through a series of steps, a cell can create C1P from other innocent fats, but the initial steps are turned on by inflammation signals. However it happens, once C1P accrues to a certain point, it flips the same switches as 4-HNE and the fat cells become limited in their ability to multiply, increasing fat cell insulin resistance.[11]

But the story isn't over. As mentioned earlier, regardless of the mechanism, we know that having more, smaller fat cells is better, metabolically speaking, than having fewer, larger fat cells.[12] For reasons including lack of insulin response and poor blood flow,[13] the larger, fewer fat cells begin leaking not only fat but also proteins called cytokines that promote inflammation (more on this in the next chapter).

As the fat cells continue belching these toxic contents into the blood, tissues "downstream" of the fat cells, including the liver and muscle, are the victims. So, in this fat-centric perspective, the fight starts in the fat cells but soon carries over to the liver and muscles (and more).

Ectopic Obesity

Fat should be stored in fat cells; this is how our bodies are built. We certainly do have a limited capacity to store fat elsewhere, but ideally this is kept at a minimum. When we store too much fat in nonfat tissues (called ectopic fat), problems arise, including insulin resistance. A few tissues appear highly relevant to this process, including the liver, pancreas, and muscles; once they become insulin resistant, the rest of the body starts to feel it.

In each of these tissues, there is a reflection of what we see in the sick fat cell—it's storing the wrong kind of fat. Triglycerides appear to be benign, even outside our fat cells. The real problems start when the fat is converted into ceramides; these "mean fats" compromise the cell's insulin functions, whether it be in the liver, pancreas, or muscle.[14]

Fatty Liver

By now, you're aware that the liver can get fat through a couple of processes, including too much fructose or alcohol or by too much insulin, which pushes the liver to create fats from carbohydrates. Regardless of the cause, when the liver starts to get fat, it starts to become insulin resistant. Once this happens, it begins releasing glucose even when it shouldn't. Generally, when insulin is high, it tells the liver to pull in and store glucose as glycogen and prevents the breakdown of glycogen back into blood glucose. Once insulin resistant, the liver allows glycogen to break down even when it shouldn't, resulting in blood glucose levels that are constantly being elevated. This creates a battle with insulin, which keeps trying to push glucose out of the blood (including into the liver), while the liver keeps dumping glucose back into the blood. This chronic battle exacerbates the insulin resistance throughout the body by ensuring insulin stays almost constantly elevated.

Fatty Pancreas

The pancreas is responsible for insulin production, so it's little surprise it's listed here. However, unlike data about the liver, the data suggesting that fatty pancreas is relevant are more tempting than they are conclusive.[15] The fatty pancreas could just be another symptom of insulin resistance and excess body fat; however, it might matter. For example, one study in China found that people with fatty pancreases were almost 60% more likely to have confirmed insulin resistance. A separate study of type 2 diabetes patients who were tracked for over two years revealed that pancreatic beta cells experienced a return to normal function around the same time that pancreas fat declined substantially. None of this is conclusive, but it may offer some valuable insight.[16]

Fatty Muscles

If the muscles become insulin resistant, it will be almost impossible to clear glucose from the blood. By mass, muscle is the largest tissue in most of our bodies and represents the largest "glucose sink"—it's the main consumer of blood glucose, and it heavily relies on insulin to open the doors to glucose and escort it into the muscle cells. As I mentioned earlier, if the muscles are just storing benign triglycerides, they seem to respond to insulin just fine[17]; again, it all depends on the type of fat it's storing. Once fat is converted to ceramides in the muscle, they start attacking several proteins in the muscle that would normally attempt to respond to insulin, effectively stopping the insulin signaling as long as the ceramides are around.

One very important aspect of insulin resistance is that muscle can become insulin resistant on its own—it doesn't need the fat cells to become insulin resistant first. Several studies have confirmed this, including studies from my own lab and others': when insulin is high for a prolonged period, muscle cells stop responding to it.[18]

LIPODYSTROPHY—TOO LITTLE OF A GOOD THING

We live in a culture that despises body fat; we do everything we can to fight it. Thus, most people would envy someone who, due to a genetic mutation, is not capable of making fat tissue. This is a condition known as lipodystrophy. However, a lack of fat tissue does not mean an inability to store fat. While the person with lipodystrophy looks as lean as you'd expect (no subcutaneous fat tissue), the body is so determined to store fat that it stores it in other tissues, including muscles and the liver. As these tissues become loaded with the ectopic fat just discussed, they become insulin resistant and create a state of severe insulin resistance in the body.[19]

Thus, rather than curse our body fat, we should be grateful for it; we might not like the way it looks, but it's healthier than the alternative.

Teasing apart insulin resistance and body fat is a challenge—they have so many varied connections. Despite conflicting evidence on which comes first, as fat cells grow, they tend to develop and promote a general resistance to insulin throughout the body. However, this doesn't mean the excess fat cell growth is obvious! Remember, "obesity" isn't a required event; sometimes the fat cell growth is relatively minor or in places that are less obvious or simply not meant for fat storage.

Throughout this chapter I've highlighted the reality that not all fats, even when stored improperly, are bad for insulin signaling. Whether a fat is nice or mean is a process of conversion—the right (or wrong) set of biochemical circumstances pushes the nice fat over the edge. Let's look at those circumstances now.

CHAPTER 12

Inflammation and Oxidative Stress

O UR POP-CULTURE UNDERSTANDING of inflammation and oxidative stress has given these two processes bad reputations. Inflammation and oxidative stress are actually two critical components of our immune system—they are there to help the body not only defend against infections but also to recover and heal when it has been damaged. In both instances, the body's primary immune cells can use inflammatory and oxidative stress events as needed to defend against invaders (such as bacteria) and help tissue repair itself.

However necessary and even occasionally beneficial these processes are, in certain circumstances, they can cross the line from good to bad, causing a cascade of events leading to the development of insulin resistance. Let's take a look.

Inflammation

Researchers first identified inflammation as a cause of insulin resistance while studying the problems that accompany infections. People with prolonged infections (which, naturally, come along with an increase in immunity-inflammation processes) develop insulin resistance.[1] This is most obviously relevant in a person who is experiencing an infection-related illness, such as infectious mononucleosis.[2] Periodontitis, which is inflammation of the gums of the mouth, can also cause insulin resistance.[3] However, inflammation and insulin resistance is also relevant in autoimmune diseases, where the body's own immune system is attacking itself. For example, the inflammatory joint disease rheumatoid arthritis, where a person's body is destroying their own joints, is heavily associated with insulin resistance to the point that those individuals who experience the worst inflammation also experience the greatest insulin resistance.[4] The same effect is seen with other inflammatory autoimmune diseases, such as lupus and Crohn's disease.[5] Even the most toxic and lethal forms of inflammation, such as sepsis, lead to insulin resistance.[6]

Revisiting Obesity (Again)

Far less serious than sepsis, though far more common, obesity is also an inflammatory disorder. As a person's fat cells grow too large, the level of immune proteins in the blood increases to the point that, in many instances, obesity is referred to as a state of chronic inflammation.[7] While inflammation is less obvious with obesity than overt inflammatory diseases like rheumatoid arthritis, its effects are nonetheless felt, even with insulin resistance. In the early 1990s, reports were published that detailed how fat tissue itself contributes to inflammation and ultimately causes insulin resistance.[8]

Fat tissue is capable of producing proteins and hormones, including inflammatory proteins called cytokines[9] (as you recall, we started to look at these in the last chapter). As cytokines are flowing from the fat tissue, something that happens more readily when fat cells are "too big" (as opposed to "too many"), they turn on inflammatory processes in cells throughout the body, especially the liver and muscles. Once inflammatory pathways are activated, innocent fats become the dangerous fats called ceramides that actively work against insulin signaling in cells.[10] Tissues where ceramide accumulates become insulin resistant.[11]

As noted, visceral fat is more harmful than subcutaneous fat. Understandably, too much fat storage surrounding our internal organs could become problematic—the fat could start to impede organ function. This is why visceral fat, pound for pound, is more inflammatory than subcutaneous fat.[12] Possibly in an effort to remove the fat from these fat cells and reduce the size of the fat, visceral fat tissue becomes populated with macrophages, the prototypical white blood cells whose main job is to clean up cellular messes. Unfortunately, as an individual continues to accrue visceral fat (due to diet and genetics), the macrophage begins to lose the battle and is itself filled with fat—becoming a "foam cell" (see pages 21–22). The foam cells send out inflammatory proteins to bring other macrophages to the area to help; they, too, will become foam cells over time, and the problem will build.

ASTHMA

Further on, we'll discuss the role of environmental toxins in causing insulin resistance (chapter thirteen). Inflammation is an important part of what causes insulin resistance when people inhale toxins, such as cigarette smoke[13]; primary and secondary smoke exposure both increase inflammation throughout the body. However, while anyone exposed to these inhaled toxins, even healthy people, will have some degree of inflammation,[14] certain people are more sensitive to them than others. These individuals may develop respiratory sensitivities such as asthma and similar complications as a result. Interestingly, these more sensitive individuals are also more likely to be insulin resistant. In both children[15] and adults,[16] asthma is highly linked to insulin resistance, which very likely develops as a result of the chronic exaggerated inflammatory response accompanying repeat exposure to inhaled toxins.[17]

In the course of just trying to do its job, inflammation inadvertently drives insulin resistance. Of course, it's pushed into it by factors outside of its control, most especially diet and, in some instances, preexisting problems, such as autoimmune disorders. Where inflammation is driving insulin resistance, it does so with the help of intermediates, like ceramides—inflammation is like the leader of a gang, and molecules like ceramides are the grunts. And oxidative stress is the head of another, albeit smaller, gang.

Oxidative Stress

"Oxidative stress" is a broad term that refers to the damage that harmful molecules cause to a cell. These dangerous molecules commonly originate from the mitochondria, the parts of the cell that use oxygen to break down glucose and fats to produce energy. This process is happening all the time. One of the products of this process is to turn oxygen into water (known as "metabolic water" because it's produced from metabolic reactions in the cell; this is why a camel doesn't need to drink water very often). It's a complicated process, but the simplified explanation is that adding a hydrogen atom and an electron onto an oxygen molecule produces water. The problem arises when the oxygen only gets an electron without a hydrogen; this is the beginning of a series of steps that produces those problematic molecules called reactive oxygen species (ROS).

This oxidative stress changes the way some proteins work in the cell, including those that insulin needs to do its job. A prevailing theory is that various proteins involved in a cell's normal response to insulin are affected and cease to function properly, reducing the cell's ability to respond to insulin.[18]

There are two sides to the oxidative-stress equation: the factors that *produce* the harmful reactive molecules and the factors that *remove* them. Exercise, for example, is a stressful event—it accelerates mitochondrial production of ROS in the working muscles. However, it also increases our ability to remove ROS. Importantly, the improved defense against ROS lingers longer than the acute, exercise-induced production of ROS. Thus, the net effect of exercise is to reduce oxidative stress.

Evidence of oxidative stress causing insulin resistance in humans is surprisingly equivocal. Insulin-resistant people do tend to have more markers of oxidative stress compared with their insulin-sensitive counterparts.[19] That isn't surprising considering that increased blood glucose and free fatty acids (as occurs with insulin resistance) boosts oxidative stress.[20] However, while several studies suggest improved insulin sensitivity with antioxidant treatment,[21] others reveal little or no benefit.[22] A problem might be the possibility that oxidative stress does not cause insulin resistance (though it might!) but merely accompanies it.

Thank heavens for inflammation and oxidative stress—our immune systems would be helpless without these two powerful weapons against infections and more. However, as a result of lifestyle and numerous unhealthy habits, these weapons are too often directed at our own bodies, resulting in chronic metabolic disruptions that ultimately drive insulin resistance. It's time to look at the various lifestyle factors (big and small) to learn how they influence insulin resistance.

CHAPTER 13

Lifestyle Factors

B Y NOW, it should be clear that our environment and how we choose to interact with that environment (whether we can control our choices or not) both play into the conditions that create insulin resistance and its effects on health. I've mentioned how foods, physical activity, medications, and substances in the environment can cause hormone changes, inflammation, obesity, and more. Now it's time to look at those factors in depth. Though these aspects cover a very broad range of topics, I think we can neatly lump them under "lifestyle factors," with a general focus on the things we *put in* our bodies and the things we *do to* our bodies.

Things We Breathe

We breathe constantly, taking roughly 20,000 breaths per day. Because of this, what we breathe can profoundly affect our health. If the air is clean, we get healthier; if it's not clean, we suffer. The incredible industrialization that has occurred in the past 150 years has exposed us to inhaled substances never seen before, and, as we'll see, that may have contributed to our rising rates of insulin resistance.

Air Pollution

The haze you see hovering over a city, or indeed an entire region, is a cocktail of several biologically active pollutants—molecules that are known to harm health. The main contributor to this haze is burning fuel, both from overtly harmful and obvious sources like our cars and power plants and subtle and seemingly innocent sources like the furnaces and water heaters in our homes.

We've known for years that air pollution is linked to insulin resistance and type 2 diabetes, according to epidemiological and intervention studies.[1] But more recently, we've explored the specific components of the air pollution that foster disease.

Perhaps the most commonly studied, and thus most implicated substance, is particulate matter up to 2.5 microns in size (known, logically enough, as PM2.5). Because of their remarkably small size, these particles are considered among the most lethal of all air pollutants—they are so small that they penetrate deeply into the lungs and are even capable of entering the blood.[2] Because PM2.5 is such a widely known breathing hazard, virtually every metropolitan area has online listings of its daily (if not hourly) levels of PM2.5. However, both PM2.5, the smallest classification of measured air pollution, and its larger counterparts (such as PM10), which can't be absorbed into the blood, are able to affect the entire body by activating inflammation.

When these toxic molecules enter the lungs, immune cells (like macrophages) sense them and activate those pro-inflammatory proteins called cytokines. As we have seen, once they're in the blood, cytokines circulate and interact with all tissues, like the liver and muscles, potentially causing them to become insulin resistant.

Cigarette Smoke

Cigarette smoke exposure damages multiple organ systems, increasing the risk of several debilitating chronic diseases, particularly cardiovascular and respiratory ones. Although US smoking rates are steadily declining, cigarette smoke is nevertheless the most common cause of preventable death. It also remains a relatively common inhaled toxin; almost half of the US population is regularly exposed to cigarette smoke,[3] and approximately 20% of young children live with a smoker in the home.[4] Worldwide, the picture is grimmer; one billion people smoke, and countless others are exposed to that smoke. And numbers outside the US are increasing, by roughly 200 million new smokers in the past 20 years. Obviously, this represents a substantial health burden.

While a great deal of attention has rightly focused on the obvious heart and lung effects with smoke exposure, cigarette smoke also profoundly desensitizes the whole body to insulin. Dr. Gerald Reaven was the first to identify a relationship between smoking and insulin resistance over 20 years ago,[5] and multiple studies since then have corroborated his findings.[6]

One of these corroborating studies warrants mention simply because of how remarkable it is. All research on cigarette smoke and insulin resistance comes from either animal interventions or studies in humans done prospectively (that is, watching for future outcomes in a current sample of participants) or retrospectively (looking at a past population for specific trends). Of course, everybody knows you can't take a group of nonsmoking people and have them smoke for a study; that would be deeply unethical. Nonetheless, without such a study we cannot *definitively* claim that smoking *causes* insulin resistance in humans. Despite the ethical questions this study raises, a group of scientists in Bulgaria was able to prove it. They took seven healthy nonsmoking people and had them smoke four cigarettes over an hour for three days.[7] Sure enough—the participants manifested insulin resistance after just their first cigarette smoke exposure. (We can only hope they didn't get hooked.)

Importantly, insulin resistance not only afflicts the actual smoker; it also raises others' resistance, through secondhand or "sidestream" smoke. In fact, work from my own lab identified that even secondhand smoke is enough to produce ceramides, those same bad fats that are likely one of the main drivers of smoke-induced insulin resistance.[8]

India and China have the dubious honor of experiencing the greatest health burden caused by massive levels of air pollution—including PM2.5 and cigarette smoke. They consistently have the worst air in the world. These countries are going through robust economic and industrial growth, which is good, but that growth has happened largely without regulations to control pollution. Interestingly, China and India are also among the countries with the greatest rates of people developing insulin resistance and type 2 diabetes.

THIRDHAND SMOKE

You know about firsthand smoke (puffing the cigarette itself) and secondhand smoke (breathing near someone who's smoking). In both instances, a person is inhaling the fumes from the burning cigarette.

However, those fumes, and the chemicals they contain, don't go away when the smoke has dissipated—they linger and stick to things, like walls, clothing, upholstery, and even hair (a win for us bald guys!). These persistent chemicals are referred to as "thirdhand" smoke—and, remarkably, they retain their ability to cause metabolic damage.[9] This lingering nature of cigarette smoke is tragically relevant to the little child, crawling along the carpet, grabbing and playing with adults' hair and clothing.

Of all the noxious chemicals one inhales from cigarette smoke, nicotine—the main addictive component—is at least part of the problem. We discussed the role of "sick fat cells" earlier; when fat cells become insulin resistant, the rest of the body often does, too. Fat cells are one of the direct sites where nicotine acts to create insulin resistance,[10] though other tissues appear to suffer the same response, such as muscle.[11]

Nowadays, there are several vehicles a person can use to get nicotine, including nicotine gum and electronic cigarettes ("e-cigs" or "vaping"), and they all increase insulin resistance. In one study that weaned cigarette smokers off smoking and onto nicotine gum, those that used the gum actually experienced a worsening of insulin resistance, whereas those that didn't use the gum had evidence of a general improvement.[12] Though the evidence is still somewhat sparse, vaping could cause similar problems.[13]

The solution to breathing dirty air, whether deliberate or accidental, is obvious, if not easy: don't breathe it—it's all or nothing, and nothing is better. However, when it comes to the food we eat, it's a little trickier; we don't need to smoke, but we do need to eat.

Things We Eat

The other common route of exposure to a harmful substance is through the mouth. Even the most diligent individual consumes harmful molecules, some of which are known to cause insulin resistance.

We'll discuss the role of diet in greater detail in chapter fifteen; before we get to that, however, it's worth mentioning some specific ingredients and ingested substances that have been particularly tied to insulin resistance.

Monosodium Glutamate

Monosodium glutamate (MSG) is still used widely due to its flavor-enhancing attributes, yet it is widely known to be harmful to health, which is why various restaurants and products are quick to advertise their food as "MSG free." Remarkably, MSG was one of the earliest-used methods of inducing obesity in lab animals![14] Needless to say, MSG increases insulin; giving people an oral load (taking in a large amount in a short time) of MSG increases the insulin response to a glucose load,[15] and every 1 gram of MSG, a daily level often reached throughout Asia, correlates with a 14% increased risk of developing insulin resistance.[16] (There are trace levels of MSG in natural foods, such as certain fruits and vegetables, though these are negligibly low.)

Petrochemicals

Petrochemicals are simply chemicals that are produced from petroleum. The number of petrochemicals is massive, encompassing thousands of commonly used items. These aren't rare, either; virtually every person on Earth uses them every day. Petrochemicals are found in items we wear, lotions we apply, and, yes, even foods we eat or drink. Most are likely inert, but at least some affect our health and even appear to influence insulin sensitivity.[17]

The main petrochemical that has been explored as a cause of insulin resistance is bisphenol A (BPA). BPA is everywhere. It is found in soft plastic water bottles and jugs, baby bottles, plastic toys, and the lining of canned foods. In the US, roughly 95% of the population has demonstrable BPA levels in the blood.[18] In animals, BPA exposure directly increases insulin resistance and insulin levels in the blood. In humans, the correlation has been robust and consistent—those with higher blood and urine BPA levels are those more likely to have insulin resistance.

Just how BPA may be causing insulin resistance is not yet fully clear. However, it might be due to its ability to imitate estrogens,[19] which, with chronic elevated levels of exposure, can induce insulin resistance.[20]

Pesticides

"Pesticide" defines a broad class of chemicals used to deter or kill insects. The use of pesticides and our subsequent exposure are both remarkable; the world uses billions of pounds annually (the US uses less than most countries). Nevertheless, like petrochemicals, pesticides are everywhere. Organochlorine (OC) pesticides (such as DDT) were once the most common type; although rarer in recent decades, their effects still linger. OC exposure has been shown to highly predict insulin resistance. One study, which followed its participants from the mid-'80s to the mid-'00s, found that those with the highest OC levels in their blood were the most likely to develop insulin resistance.[21] Shorter-term studies have since corroborated these findings.[22]

BPA and OCs are alike in how they linger. Our bodies have a remarkable ability to retain these toxins—they're gifts that just keep giving. Once we've been exposed, our bodies will often store these harmful foreign molecules in our fat tissue. Someone already carrying more fat thus likely has a greater capacity to store these toxins. And visceral fat is much more likely to accumulate these toxins—potentially up to 10 times more than subcutaneous fat.[23]

Sugar and Artificial Sweeteners

By now, you know that sugar influences insulin. Our increasing consumption of sweetened foods—products with added natural sugars or high-fructose corn syrup—has unsurprisingly coincided with rising rates of insulin resistance.

Fructose has become frighteningly prevalent. It's found in a remarkable number of processed and packaged foods (~70%), whether as pure fructose, sucrose (which is glucose + fructose), or high-fructose corn syrup. Increasingly, pure fructose is used even in "health" products, from sports drinks to protein powders. Many people assume it to be a "natural ingredient" and, therefore, healthier than sugar and other sweeteners. An interesting trend with fructose (and its various forms) is how widely used it continues to be with little thought of the consequences.

Regardless of its source, whether pure (e.g., crystallized fructose) or in combination (e.g., sucrose), fructose has been shown to increase insulin resistance.[24] The exact way this works isn't definite; it might be through its effects on body fat storage (as we discussed when we talked about liver health—see page 72) or by increasing inflammation.[25]

Earlier, we spoke about oxidative stress. Sugar, which is half glucose and half fructose, increases oxidative stress quite readily.[26] Of course, this combination of simple carbohydrates increases blood glucose and insulin—the higher it gets, the greater the oxidative stress.[27]

Artificial sweeteners are a broad class of non-nutritive compounds—things that taste like sugar but provide few or no calories and no nutrition. The evidence on specific sweeteners and insulin resistance is sparse, though there is enough to mention.

Researchers have concluded that artificial sweeteners increase the *risk* of insulin resistance. According to one study, people who drink an artificially sweetened (diet) soda daily have a 36% greater chance of developing metabolic syndrome and a whopping 67% higher risk of type 2 diabetes.[28] These studies are correlational and, thus, prevent us from making any real conclusions about sweeteners and insulin resistance. However, the strong correlation does hint at a causal connection. A few theories might explain it, including that artificial sweeteners increase our craving for "real" food,[29] trick us into thinking we can eat more later (i.e., "Because this soda doesn't have any calories, I can eat these fries"),[30] and (my favorite) may cause a small insulin spike[31] even though they provide no meaningful calories.

Let's unpack this last one a bit. This phenomenon is known as the cephalic phase insulin response (CPIR), and it's a natural reaction to sweet foods that helps prepare the body for a carbohydrate load. Because it should! In nature, anything that tastes sweet would be a carbohydrate. The CPIR is simply the body's way of "priming the pump" by releasing a little insulin in anticipation of a carbohydrate load, which will cause a greater insulin release later. One interesting study explored the effects of various sweeteners on altering the insulin release from eating. Each subject drank one of various sweetened drinks with a meal.[32] Drinking sucrose (sugar) with the meal had the highest effect on insulin release, but, interestingly, aspartame consumption with the meal had an almost identical effect to sugar (though there is evidence to challenge this[33]). Stevia, erythritol, and monk fruit extract, however, had no effect.

Keep in mind that these data are focused on drinking a sweetener *while eating a meal*; consuming the sweeteners on their own appears to do nothing.[34]

NON-NUTRITIVE TO US, BUT NUTRITIVE TO OUR BACTERIA?

There is evidence to support the idea that sweeteners affect gut bacteria (not necessarily in a bad way),[35] and this possible alteration could explain how some sweeteners can affect glucose and insulin levels in some people but not others.[36] Again, these are all theories, but if the gut-bacteria perspective is valid, the effects of sweeteners, very frustratingly, could depend on the person.

Lipopolysaccharides

Before concluding this section, I want to include a final contestant for what may be considered the worst toxin. Lipopolysaccharides (LPS) are molecules that are inherently part of a certain type of bacteria and are known to activate very specific immune events in the body.

What's remarkable about LPS is that it is everywhere; in the food we eat, the water we drink, and even, in some instances, the air we breathe.[37] Thus, LPS is a toxin that fits under both inhaled and ingested toxins. LPS research is intimately connected to the flourishing research done over the past 10 years into the role of gut bacteria and metabolic disruption like insulin resistance.

Similar to the previously mentioned toxins, LPS activates an inflammatory response, which involves inflammatory proteins moving throughout the entire circulatory system (and, as we know, inflammation is connected to insulin resistance). However, LPS *itself* is detectable in the blood—and, indeed, in higher amounts in the blood of overweight and insulin-resistant individuals.[38] Yet we don't know just how or why LPS is able to get from the gut or lungs into the blood. Some evidence indicates that LPS is more readily absorbed from the gut when we eat particular nutrients, such as fat[39] or fructose.[40] However, these conclusions are limited, as the majority of research on this topic has been done with rodents, which respond very differently to foods and LPS than humans.

LDL CHOLESTEROL: OUR DEFENSE AGAINST LPS

Cholesterol and its lipoprotein carriers (HDL, LDL, and VLDL) are too often discussed in negative terms, as if they're something to fear. However, these lipoproteins, especially LDL, also play an important role in "neutralizing" LPS. Specifically, they carry a protein called "LPS-binding protein." As you might guess, it physically binds the LPS and escorts it to the liver, passing from there into the intestines and out of the body.[41] In fact, this may be why people with lower LDL cholesterol levels are more likely to experience severe infections.[42]

Too Little Salt

No, that's not a typo—eating too little salt can create metabolic problems. Because of the fear that salt may increase blood pressure (though it depends on the person; see page 15), medical practitioners have been recommending for decades that we eat less salt. The thought is that getting too little salt is better than the risk of consuming too much. Unfortunately, this is simply incorrect.

In one study, researchers took 27 men with normal or elevated blood pressure and restricted their salt intake for one week.[43] The first piece of bad news: their blood pressure did not drop. Even worse: they became insulin resistant. It's no wonder the authors felt inclined to note the "potentially adverse impact of dietary salt restriction." An additional study corroborated the observation that too little salt results in insulin resistance: 152 healthy men and women had alternating weeks of low- or high-salt diets, with insulin levels and insulin resistance measured at the end of each week.[44] Similar to the previous study, subjects became significantly more insulin resistant when they ate less salt.

The explanation for this salt-sensitive response is based on hormones. As salt consumption drops, the kidneys initiate a process to reabsorb as much as salt as possible from the urine back into the blood. Remember, this happens through the actions of aldosterone (for a refresher, turn back to page 15). However, while aldosterone is working to recover urinary salt, it also antagonizes insulin, creating insulin resistance.[45]

Starvation

"Eat less" has been a staple of conventional thinking with regard to controlling glucose and insulin for people who are overweight and have type 2 diabetes.

Unfortunately, while it's partly based in evidence, this vague advice can potentially be misapplied or outright abused; there is a fine line between fasting and starving. Eating too little for too long can become harmful, as is the case with eating disorders, such as anorexia nervosa or bulimia nervosa. What's more, as we've seen, there are remarkable and unexpected effects on children born to mothers in conditions of chronic food deprivation; see pages 39–40.

An important distinction between fasting, even multiday fasts, and starvation is the state of muscle tissue. If a fast continues to the point of demonstrable muscle loss, the gap has officially been crossed: fasting has turned into starvation. This isn't something that happens very readily—we're aren't good for much if we have too little muscle to move our bodies. The body defends muscle until we run low on fat—and because we all have varying levels of body fat, it's difficult to put a definite number of days to when we cross that gap.

Still, done right, fasting can be an effective strategy to manage insulin levels. We'll discuss the therapeutic use of intermittent fasting in chapter fifteen.

Things We Do

Separate from the food we eat or the air we breathe, our daily acts of living matter a great deal to our metabolic health and insulin sensitivity. These things we do are varied, of course—we all have different lives and daily tasks—but we all share a couple that matter a great deal for maintaining healthy insulin function.

Sleep

When we sleep, our responsiveness to the environment is dialed down, allowing our bodies to recover. We all know getting enough sleep is necessary for good health. (New parents be warned: you won't enjoy reading this . . .) But how do we define "enough" when it comes to sleep?

The classic story is that we all need around eight hours per night of meaningful sleep, but this isn't necessarily the case. Very recent evidence suggests that multiple earlier cultures were early to rise . . . or late to bed. On average, it appears that our ancestors likely slept from five to seven hours at night, less than today's recommended eight hours. It's possible that some of us may simply need less sleep than others. Some of us have a mutation in a gene (*DEC2*) that allows us to thrive on substantially little sleep.[46]

While we can debate the actual ideal length of time for nightly sleep, there is a very clear, scientifically supported consensus that not getting enough sleep, whatever that may mean for each individual, is harmful to health. One of potentially many negative effects of developing a sleep debt is pronounced changes in the endocrine system— our hormones change. In particular, just one week of less sleep can make the body roughly 30% more insulin resistant compared with a week of normal sleep.[47] In fact, a very recent study suggests this effect is even more potent; just two days of sleep restriction (~50% of normal) was enough to make otherwise healthy men insulin resistant.[48]

TOO MUCH LIGHT IS A HEAVY MATTER

If a person struggles with insomnia, it may not matter so much they're awake more at night, but rather what they do when they're awake at night. Specifically, being exposed to bright lights, such as the glow of a small electronic screen, may be the determining factor of whether or not a person develops insulin resistance with sleep deprivation. Exposure to light at night alters our levels of melatonin and, importantly, cortisol; this effect isn't as great during sleep deprivation *without* light exposure, suggesting that remaining in the dark potentially mediates the insulin resistance.[49]

Given that sleep deprivation can lead to insulin resistance, who would have thought that napping too much could cause a problem with it, as well? As with nightly sleep, time matters. With napping, the magic number appears to be around 30 minutes. Compared with non-nappers, those who nap more than roughly one hour each day are more likely to develop insulin resistance, whereas those who nap up to 30 minutes each day are less likely to develop it.[50]

Sedentary Living

The maxim "use it or lose it" could apply to insulin sensitivity and physical activity—the less we move our body, the more insulin resistant it becomes. In fact, this phenomenon is so widely observed and strong that many suspect physical inactivity is a main reason why insulin resistance tends to worsen with age.[51] Being sedentary for a few days causes demonstrable insulin resistance even in otherwise healthy people,[52] and the problem only gets worse in older people.[53] And this isn't a subtle effect—just one week of being sedentary can increase insulin resistance sevenfold![54] In fact, a few weeks of immobility has a lasting effect with insulin resistance; even when a person becomes mobile again, the insulin resistance persists for weeks at around double what it would be in a person who maintained physical activity.

Insulin resistance through disuse is mostly a result of our muscles: because we don't use them, they respond less to insulin. Interestingly, the insulin resistance occurs with incredible precision, based on the muscles that are not being used. For example, if one leg is in a cast (and thus immobile), that leg becomes half as insulin sensitive as the mobile leg within just days.[55] The molecular mechanisms that explain the insulin resistance in the immobile muscle are fascinating—essentially, the immobility hijacks the inflammation pathways. We've explored how inflammation can cause insulin resistance (see chapter twelve), and those same events occur in the case of disuse: the unused muscle experiences an increase in activity of inflammatory events, which drive the insulin resistance.[56]

Even something as seemingly benign as sitting for too long, too often, is associated with greater insulin resistance.[57] A very interesting study found that by having people sit for two hours prior to a meal, versus occasionally interrupting the sitting, the blood glucose response to a meal was roughly 45% higher.[58] The simple solution to buffering the harm on insulin resistance of sitting is to simply break it up roughly every 20 minutes for as little as two minutes. For instance, just flex your muscles from time to time; contracting a muscle 30 times for a few seconds each is enough to help reduce the risk.[59]

I know what you're thinking: there are so many things to worry about in life, and now we have to worry about the air we breathe, the chemicals we swallow, and more. While it's impossible to get all this 100% right, we should make an effort to genuinely scrutinize our habits and our environments to determine the variables we can control. If you live in a city with horrible air quality, you can't change that; you might consider purchasing a breathing mask that can filter PM2.5. Sleep, as elusive as it is, gets better as good habits are practiced—especially getting off screens well before bedtime.

I hope you've highlighted some aspects of your environment and behaviors that you can focus on. The sum of these small efforts is larger than the individual parts; as inconsequential as each might seem, putting away your phone earlier in the evening and more frequently replacing your home air filter will affect how your body senses and responds to insulin. But you'll want to do much more after you learn further solutions to preventing and reversing insulin resistance—and that's what we'll discuss in the next part of this book.

PART III

The Solution
How Can We Fight
Insulin Resistance?

CHAPTER 14

Get Moving:
The Importance of
Physical Activity

HAVING THOROUGHLY COVERED the causes of—and the many diseases and disorders that arise from—insulin resistance, it's time for the happy ending: there are multiple avenues available for preventing and even reversing it. The goal of this section is to highlight findings that are scientifically supported to improve insulin resistance, while conveying the benefits and, where relevant, the drawbacks.

I am a firm believer that changing the way we live can effectively cut our risk of developing insulin resistance and even remove it after we've developed the disorder. I am aware that such a paradigm can be both discouraging and empowering; making a commitment to change your exercise regimen or your diet is not as easy as taking a pill, and the results are not as rapid as those following bariatric surgery. However, by changing the way we live, we can address the fundamental origins of what's occurring in the body to cause insulin resistance in the first place, rather than treat symptoms through drugs or undergo dramatic, often irreversible surgical procedures (as we'll see in chapter sixteen).

Thus, how we live can be both the culprit of and the cure for insulin resistance. Of course, as we saw earlier, there are various factors, such as genetics and environmental pollution, over which we have little to no control. But for the overwhelming majority of people, including almost every person reading this—and that means you!—we can control how we live. And even if other insulin-resistance factors (like our genes) aren't in our favor, lifestyle is the most powerful change we can make.

The two essential components of lifestyle that encompass the risks of insulin resistance are how we move and what we eat—in other words, exercise and diet.

Before you groan at the lack of originality in this statement and before you put your head in your hands in fear of the perceived discipline and patience required, know that changing your physical activity and the foods you eat does not need to be the harrowing experience you might have undergone before. In the context of insulin resistance (and the many diseases stemming from it), when it comes to diet and exercise, what you think you know may be wrong . . . and what you might have tried before probably wasn't as helpful as you thought. So no more training for a marathon you may never run (or walk), and it's time to put away the fat-free foods.

Movement Matters

Exercise is very helpful for improving insulin resistance. In fact, any kind of physical activity can help to combat insulin resistance because it removes glucose from the blood without involving insulin.

A bit of review might be helpful. Back in chapter one, I told you that insulin "'opens the doors' to escort glucose from the blood to various parts of the body, such as the brain, heart, muscles, and fat tissue." Our bodies rely on insulin to usher glucose from the blood into these tissues and get our levels back to normal. In fact, this clearance process is so vital, that the main glucose eaters, our muscles, can get the glucose for themselves.

To move our body in any way, we must contract (flex) muscles. Interestingly, as muscles contract, they are able to take in glucose from the blood *without* using insulin. (As an aside, there is a myth that muscle uses only glucose for energy. Muscle can indeed use other fuel sources, like fat or ketones, perfectly well—and you'll understand in a few pages why I mention this.) This means that even if a muscle is resistant to insulin, it can still pull glucose from the bloodstream when contracting. Because movement enables this insulin-independent process, our blood insulin naturally lowers during and shortly after exercise.[1] In fact, just moving is so helpful that the body becomes more insulin sensitive even in the absence of any weight changes.[2]

Other than muscle contraction and the insulin-bypass process involved with it, exercise appears to improve insulin sensitivity by easing many of its causes, such as central obesity, oxidative stress, inflammation, and more. One study had insulin-resistant individuals engage in moderate-intensity walking for three months.[3] Even over the course of the relatively brief study, the people lost an average of 2% body fat, which appeared to largely come from visceral fat. A 2% change isn't much, yet it was still enough to improve participants' insulin sensitivity. Moreover, another study found that a three-month exercise intervention reduced markers of inflammation and oxidative stress in the absence of weight loss.[4] Regular and even light exercise can also improve sleep and may reduce markers of stress.[5]

EXERCISE AND WEIGHT LOSS

With how much you hear about exercise and body weight, you might expect a near consensus from research that exercise leads to significant weight loss.

Interestingly, decades of data make it clear: exercise alone is not an effective intervention for weight loss.[6] Yet this certainly isn't a reason to *not* exercise—the benefits of exercise may not include weight loss, but do include several others, including stronger muscles and bones and better-functioning heart and lungs.

Another interesting aspect of exercise as an intervention to improve insulin resistance is that it works across all ages and sexes.[7] In one study, just 16 weeks of regular exercise not only improved strength by almost 50% in men aged 50 to 65, but also increased their insulin sensitivity by over 20%. This was in the absence of any changes in diet—they just started exercising.

Aerobic Versus Resistance Exercise

To run (or bike or swim) or lift—that is the question.

If you have time, you can certainly do both aerobic and resistance exercise; you'd experience more robust improvements than you would doing either cardio or weight training alone. But in the end, most of us devote our limited hours only to the activity that yields the greatest benefit.

The overwhelming majority of research has explored the issue of exercise and insulin resistance in the context of aerobic exercise alone. However, plenty of studies have indeed confirmed that doing resistance exercise, even just twice per week, is enough to improve insulin sensitivity.[8] All of this serves to strengthen the role of regular exercise in fighting insulin resistance.

Studies that have compared the insulin-sensitizing effect of both aerobic and resistance exercise reveal that, minute for minute, resistance training may be superior in improving insulin sensitivity.[9] One study tracked roughly 32,000 people for almost 20 years and found that engaging in either aerobic or resistance exercise for 2.5 hours per week yielded similar improvements, but that resistance training was superior when the participants spent less time engaging in exercise[10] (so, if you have only one hour in a week to exercise, resistance training will have a higher return on investment). This is very likely a result of the respective changes in muscle mass that accompany each type of exercise[11]; resistance training increases muscle mass while aerobic does not.[12] You'll recall that in the average individual, muscle is the largest organ in the body; muscle is also the largest destination for insulin-stimulated glucose uptake. If we have more muscle, we have a greater area into which we can deposit glucose from the blood, thus lowering blood insulin.

BODY WEIGHT—NOT THE WHOLE STORY

Certain studies show greater improvements in body weight with aerobic exercise over resistance exercise. Of course, a lot depends on how long the study subjects exercise, which varies greatly between studies, but the larger problem with such conclusions is that body weight is not an indicator of body composition. Muscle weighs more than fat. Inasmuch as resistance exercise increases muscle mass more than aerobic exercise does, this naturally affects body weight.

To sum this up: the best exercise is the one you'll do. There is certainly a value to challenging yourself to do something you're not familiar (or even comfortable) with. However, if your dislike for one form of exercise is substantial enough that committing to it would mean you stop doing anything, stick with something you know you'll do. Just do it harder.

Intensity

Other than simply exercising regularly, the next most important variable in regard to exercise and insulin resistance is intensity. People are often quite casual about their exercise; whether it's aerobic or resistance, many of us tend to just go through the motions. Exercise should be a fairly strenuous ordeal. The effort and focus you devote to it might be unpleasant for some of us, but know that the payoff is great. Individuals who are able to exercise more vigorously have greater improvements in insulin sensitivity (and many other benefits).[13] However, if such intensity is too daunting to consider, remember that simply doing it at any intensity is the best place to begin.

THINK BEFORE YOU DRINK

If your reason for exercising is to improve your metabolic health by improving insulin sensitivity, put down the post-workout sports drink– it's making things worse. Exercise is a good way to improve insulin sensitivity. However, by adding a glucose load after your workout, which many believe is essential, you lose some of the insulin-sensitizing improvements of the exercise.[14] The best bet is to avoid sugary drinks and food for as long after the workout as you're comfortable.

In the case of aerobic exercise, a case can be made for lower-intensity workouts, especially if you're in the early stages of changing your diet; if you've started eating more fat and fewer carbs (more on that in the coming chapters), going easy on the exercise gives your body time to adapt to this alternate fuel source. With lower-intensity exercise, the body does use relatively more fat as fuel.[15] Importantly, as an individual becomes increasingly more trained, the body is able to predominantly use fat, rather than glucose, at higher and higher intensities.

As you become adapted to using fat to fuel your exercise, increasing intensity may mean a faster walk than normal, a brisk walk with intermittent sprints, a vigorous jog, or a jog with periodic sprints. The same general principle applies to any other aerobic exercise, such as cycling or swimming. In fact, for those pressed for time, simply increasing the intensity over a shorter time (~20 minutes) is at least as effective at improving insulin resistance as lower-intensity, longer duration exercise.[16] This style of exercise, termed high-intensity interval training (HIIT), is effective enough that its popularity has exploded; chances are you or someone you know is already doing it.

For resistance exercise, a higher-intensity workout means approaching or going to failure on each set, whether by increasing weight or doing more repetitions. This style of exercise not only requires some time to adjust to the more demanding routine, but it also requires greater determination—continuing with an exercise until you can't do another rep is as exhausting physically as it is mentally. Again, this isn't something one just starts doing. To avoid injury, this should be a gradual process of getting to the point where failure happens anywhere between around five to 15 repetitions. But the number of times you perform the exercise is less important than going to failure.

After reading this chapter, you might conclude that the mantra is "go often and go hard." A better takeaway would be "just do it"—start where you are by doing what you can. If you're honest with yourself (or you trust someone to be honest with you), you'll make sure you're regularly increasing either the frequency or intensity to help maximize the insulin-sensitizing effect of your efforts. Whatever you decide, and as effective as exercise can be at fighting insulin resistance, it's best matched with changes in what and when we eat.

COOL DOWN

Could our comfortable thermoneutral environments be part of our metabolic decline? Frequent exposure to cold is perhaps the most unexpected (and unpleasant) thing you can do to improve and control your insulin levels.

Before diving into the evidence suggesting cold exposure improves insulin sensitivity, I need to introduce you to a type of fat you've possibly never heard of: brown fat. Most of the fat we have on our bodies is "white fat," called "white adipose tissue" or WAT—the tissue itself is quite white, partly due to the lack of mitochondria within the fat cells (mitochondria have a brownish-red color). However, there are distinct small pockets of fat in the body where the fat cells are not only much smaller, but also very richly brown; they're loaded with mitochondria. Mitochondria are important "energy centers," making fuel for the cell by breaking down glucose and fats. However, the mitochondria in brown adipose tissue (BAT) behave a little differently from most. Generally, mitochondria will only burn nutrients (that is, carbs or fats) dependent on the energy needs of the cell; thus, the cell's energy demand determines, or is *coupled* to, cell energy production. Makes sense. However, BAT mitochondria are enriched with *uncoupling* proteins; as the name suggests, these proteins allow the mitochondria to burn nutrients and, rather than giving the cell energy, they simply produce heat. So white fat wants to store fat and brown fat wants to burn fat. In fact, when activated, BAT has a metabolic rate comparable to muscle and uses as much glucose as muscle cells.[17]

This is where the cold comes in; BAT becomes activated when our skin gets cold.

The "magic temperature" against the skin appears to be about 64.4°F (18°C)—at this temperature, BAT becomes active in men and women and starts burning glucose in an effort to warm the body.[18] This temperature is unique because, for most people, it requires the body to work a little harder to stay warm, but not work too hard. The muscles won't shiver because the BAT is able to activate and generate sufficient heat. (In fact, it's this process that explains why babies don't shiver—they have a lot of BAT that keeps them warm.) However, when the temperature drops below this point, the body begins shivering, which is a more dramatic (and effective) method of generating heat to maintain internal body temperature.

Relevant to both of these processes (shivering and nonshivering thermogenesis) is the fuel—glucose. In both processes, glucose is being consumed more rapidly than normal. Of course, the upside to this is that insulin levels drop as glucose is used. Partly because of increased glucose use by shivering muscle and activated BAT, insulin secretion drops quickly in the cold.[19]

With cold exposure, a very interesting additional change occurs in fat tissue that influences insulin sensitivity. Fat tissue is capable of producing hormones, termed adipokines, that affect myriad metabolic processes. One of the beneficial hormones that increases insulin sensitivity is adiponectin, released from WAT. Interestingly, adiponectin levels rise with cold exposure (two hours).[20]

CHAPTER 15

Eat Smart:
The Evidence on
the Food We Eat

W E HAVE NOW ARRIVED at what is the most powerful part of the
solution in the fight against insulin resistance: the food we eat.
The most powerful but also the most difficult to change. So much
has been written about this in recent decades, so for me, exploring
the benefits to insulin sensitivity as a consequence of altering the diet
required a thoughtful and deliberate analysis of published research.
The results of such an analysis led me to one unavoidable conclusion:
when it comes to diet, we got it wrong.

The epidemics of obesity and insulin resistance are partly the
product of bending science to fit politics. As documented thoroughly
by Gary Taubes (*Good Calories, Bad Calories*) and Nina Teicholz (*The
Big Fat Surprise)*, in the 1950s and 1960s, a political consensus was
created from the limited (and highly debated) data suggesting dietary
fat, particularly saturated fat, correlated with heart disease. In remarkably little time, this correlation became considered causation, and a
tentative theory become dietary dogma. Soon, we collectively learned
to vilify dietary fat as the leading cause of heart disease, weight gain,
and diabetes, though at the time the scientific community widely criti-
cized this move.

At its simplest, the battle of thought between political agenda and
scientific process centered around the relevance of calorie number versus calorie type in determining the ideal nutrition for good health. Sup-
porters of calorie number argue that it's all a matter of mathematics:
if you eat fewer calories than you expend, you'll be lean and insulin

sensitive; if you eat more calories than you expend, you'll be fat and insulin resistant. On the other side, many argue that the type of calorie is more relevant than the number; a nutrient, once consumed, affects the body's hormones, particularly insulin, and it's this subsequent insulin effect that drives insulin resistance, fat gain, and eventually disease.

Depending on your school of thought, then, the solution to insulin resistance is either restricting calories, which almost invariably means a low-fat diet, or restricting certain types of carbohydrates, which aims to keep insulin low. Now, I mentioned earlier that the human body is somewhat more complicated than a simple furnace, and there's more to diet than "calories in, calories out." Let's take a look at the research on these varied approaches.

Limiting Calories

The most common dietary intervention in our society to prevent weight gain or aid weight loss is calorie restriction, and this same tool is used in attempts to fix insulin resistance. However, whereas calorie restriction will cause weight loss, if only in the short term, its effects on insulin resistance are less conclusive.

These paradoxical findings may be explained by the type of weight that's lost. One of the problems with calorie restriction is that you have no control over where on the body the weight loss occurs. We certainly want to lower body fat. But in this state of (hopefully) mild starvation known diplomatically as calorie restriction, the body is also reducing the amount of lean mass a person has, including muscle and bone.[1] It's easy to see the problem: the less lean mass a person has, especially muscle, the less insulin-sensitive tissue is available to help clear glucose from the blood and restore insulin levels to baseline. Yes—caloric restriction can cause insulin resistance.

ANOREXIA AND INSULIN RESISTANCE

Anorexia nervosa (AN) is a condition where a person seeks an unhealthily low level of body fat through severe calorie restriction. In the "excess fat = insulin resistance" paradigm, a person with AN should be highly insulin sensitive. Unfortunately, that's not the case. Patients with AN are regularly found to be less glucose tolerant and more insulin resistant than healthy lean individuals.[2] In this scenario, "fasting" has turned into "starvation."

One remarkable study explored the metabolic consequences of strict and severe caloric restriction in obese individuals with no prior history or evidence of insulin resistance.[3] The subjects self-restricted their intake to around 800 calories a day, which resulted in varying levels of weight loss; subjects lost between 8 and 35 kilograms, or about 17 and 77 pounds. (No, 800 calories a day is not much food!) In contrast to the link between body weight and insulin resistance, this state of weight loss caused over half of the study subjects to develop insulin resistance to the point of type 2 diabetes! In fact, with severe caloric restriction, the body can become demonstrably insulin resistant in just a few days.

Very-low-calorie diets elicit stress on the body, evident in the marked changes in hormone levels, with the most prominent change being a significant increase in the quintessential stress hormone cortisol.[4] Remember, one of cortisol's main hormonal actions (as part of our fight-or-flight response with adrenaline) is to counter insulin and increase blood glucose. But cortisol's antagonistic relationship with insulin extends beyond just trying to increase glucose; cortisol actually makes the muscles (and other tissue) insulin resistant. Furthermore, thyroid levels plummet, which, in addition to lowering metabolic rate, exacerbates the problem; thyroid hormone maintains normal insulin signaling. Thus, the drop in thyroid hormones further shifts the body to an insulin-resistant state.[5]

Despite these frightening findings with severe and prolonged caloric restriction, *mild* caloric restriction, including low-fat diets, can clearly improve insulin sensitivity.[6] However, the results are sometimes not overly dramatic. As an example, in looking at the effects of 14 weeks of a low-fat, plant-based diet in overweight middle-aged women, insulin sensitivity was no different from that of participants eating the control diet.[7]

CARBS COME LAST

If you have a dietary obsession with certain carbohydrates, such as rice or pasta, and know you can't live without them, the good news is that you can use a simple trick to lessen the insulin impact: eat them at the end of your meal. In a study comparing breaking up the parts of a meal into the primary starch, protein, and vegetables, eating the starchy part of the meal after the protein and vegetables had a significantly smaller effect on blood glucose and insulin.[8]

Dietary Fiber

A low-fat, low-calorie diet is almost always going to be high in dietary fiber (that is, if it's done right, by focusing on real foods rather than processed diet meals). Dietary fiber has a special place in the hallowed halls of the nutritional pantheon; it is almost universally embraced as being essential to a modern healthy diet. Despite the many reported benefits, the role of fiber in insulin sensitivity is open to interpretation; there's a general indication that fiber improves it. Multiple epidemiological studies (that is, studies that get data from questionnaires) find a correlation between fiber consumption and improved insulin sensitivity.[9] Results from clinical trials are mixed; interpreting the results requires some scrutiny in the context of insulin resistance. Because clinical trials, not questionnaires, help establish cause and effect, we'll only focus on those.

Some studies have found that when study subjects eat a high-fiber meal, glucose and insulin levels are lower than those of subjects who eat a low-fiber meal—but again, these findings vary based on the subject population. For example, men with higher fasting insulin levels (i.e., insulin-resistant men) enjoyed a lower post-meal insulin spike when consuming a high-fiber meal versus a low-fiber meal, but there was no difference in insulin levels in the men with normal fasting insulin (i.e., insulin-sensitive men). When explored over the long term, the results get even more confusing. While increasing dietary fiber over a period of several weeks was shown to improve insulin sensitivity in a group of nonobese people with diabetes,[10] consuming more dietary fiber had no effect on insulin resistance in obese people with diabetes.[11] Altogether, these studies suggest an insulin-sensitizing effect of fiber in insulin-resistant subjects, if not insulin-sensitive subjects, and provide evidence of a possible limit to the benefits.

An important weakness in these studies is the type of fiber used. Virtually every dietary fiber trial uses fiber supplements in the form of guar gum, which is not a fiber that comes with most carbohydrates. While guar gum is available in health food stores, it is not part of a normal diet, which suggests the results of a high-fiber diet in the form of higher guar gum intake should not be extrapolated to assume that other sources of fiber like vegetables and legumes will have the same results.[12] Nevertheless, placing insulin-resistant individuals on a high-fiber diet (50 g/day) where the fiber is primarily from fruits, vegetables, legumes, and select grains, significantly improved insulin sensitivity after six weeks.[13]

An unfortunate aspect of almost every study exploring the role of dietary fiber in insulin resistance is that the study increases fiber at the expense of fat—the high-fiber study diets are low-fat diets. As we will see shortly, dietary fat elicits no effect on blood insulin, so the relative absence of fat in the high-fiber diets leaves unanswered the question of whether or not a diet high in fat *and* fiber is more effective than a diet high in fiber and low in fat. An alternative perspective is that dietary fiber is increasingly more essential as dietary carbohydrates, particularly processed, are increasingly part of the diet. Two published reports touch on this conflict, albeit without actually addressing insulin resistance, and focus on only the glucose response. One study gave participants three distinct types of bread—low fiber/low fat, high fiber/low fat, and high fiber/high fat.[14] The low fiber/low fat bread resulted in a far greater blood glucose response than the other two and was the least satisfying (suggesting that perhaps the person would be inclined to eat more). Whereas the blood glucose response was similar between the two high-fiber breads—regardless of fat content—the high-fiber/high-fat bread was more *satisfying*. Unfortunately, the study did not assess insulin levels, which prevents any conclusions touching on insulin resistance directly. A second study fed subjects four types of pasta meals—normal pasta, pasta with psyllium (fiber), pasta with fat (oil), and pasta with psyllium and fat.[15] Psyllium alone did nothing to mitigate the insulin or glucose effects of the carbohydrate-rich pasta.

While adding fat lowered them somewhat, adding both psyllium and fat lowered them the most and led to the greatest satiety.

In the end, it's very likely that fiber improves insulin sensitivity in most people by simply replacing sugars and starches that elicit an insulin response. Importantly, one should scrutinize the source of fiber; it's dumbfounding, but true, that most fiber supplements have sugar as one of the main ingredients.

Depending on the degree to which the fiber dissolves in water, dietary fiber can be defined as "soluble" (mixes well with water) or "insoluble" (does not mix well with water). Beyond their solubility, dietary fiber can be defined by its ability to benefit glucose and insulin control. Here, soluble fiber wins. Whereas insoluble fiber, derived mainly from grains and bran, provides bulk for stool, it's the soluble fiber, generally from fruits and certain vegetables (including the psyllium husk in the pasta experiments I just mentioned), or specific supplements, that provides the best glucose and insulin benefits.[16]

Intermittent Fasting or Time-Restricted Feeding

The timing of meals is an important topic, as most people are eating more frequently now than ever before. In fact, just about 30 years ago, most adults and children had daily meals separated by almost five hours, whereas today this number is down to about three and a half hours, and this doesn't include snacking between meals, something that generally didn't occur in the 1980s.[17]

A common thread among many dietary plans is when and how often to eat. The advice varies; some approaches involve compressing periods of eating to two or three meals per day, with substantial gaps in between, while other strategies suggest eating normally for a few days, then avoiding food entirely for a day. On the other end of the spectrum, some diets encourage "grazing," eating six to eight small meals per day—the antithesis of time-restricted eating.

As you now know, when we eat a meal (and especially certain foods, which we'll get into later), our blood insulin rises to control glucose levels. Because elevated insulin is one of the most relevant factors in developing insulin resistance, it makes sense to follow a dietary plan that incorporates periods of time throughout the day when insulin is kept low. So right away, you've probably guessed that more frequent eating isn't effective at controlling insulin.

When looking at the data on timing of eating, two factors become relevant—how the person eats day to day and month to month. On a larger time scale, patients who fast (for 24 hours) roughly once monthly are about half as likely to be insulin resistant compared with those who don't.[18] At the shorter end, within each day, eating fewer, larger meals elicits a greater improvement than eating several smaller meals throughout the day.[19] Very likely, the insulin benefit in eating fewer meals in the day is simply a consequence of having longer periods of time when glucose and insulin are normal in between meals. If you have more frequent meals, insulin levels would increase every couple of hours, regardless of how much you eat. If three large meals per day is better than six small ones, are fewer meals than three best of all? Possibly.

Fasting involves eating normally for some period of time, with strategic periods of food avoidance; no need to count calories. There is evidence to show fasting is effective at improving insulin sensitivity, though it partly depends on how it's done. Two studies looked at intermittent fasting by having study subjects eat normally one day and essentially fast the entire next day, repeated seven times over a two-week period. The two studies found conflicting results: one reported an improvement in insulin sensitivity,[20] while the other observed no benefit.[21] By contrast, a recent study on the use of intermittent fasting in insulin-treated people with type 2 diabetes found that frequent (a few times weekly) 24-hour fasts were so effective at improving insulin sensitivity that participants were able to cease insulin use—it was "deprescribed."[22] In fact, for one person, it happened in only five days! The alternative strategy is to confine eating to a specific window of time each day, so you'd end up eating breakfast and lunch only[23] or lunch and dinner only.[24] In these time-restricted eating studies, participants saw robust improvements in insulin sensitivity.

It may sound strange, but many of the benefits of fasting are caused by changes in hormones. Of course, insulin drops quickly with a fast, but insulin's "opposite," glucagon, rises. It's important to understand glucagon to truly appreciate the power of a fast. Where insulin tries to save energy in the body, glucagon wants to spend it—they are two sides of the same metabolic coin. Glucagon wants the body to release its stored energy by pushing the fat cells to share their fat and the liver to share its glucose. Because insulin and glucagon work against each other to activate and inhibit metabolic processes (see the diagram below), the balance of these two hormones dictates which processes actually occur. Thus, looking at fasting, and even eating, through the lens of the insulin:glucagon ratio is very helpful.

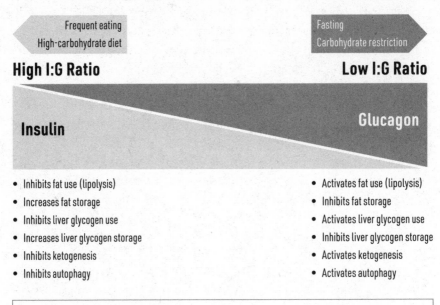

Frequent eating High-carbohydrate diet	Fasting Carbohydrate restriction
High I:G Ratio	**Low I:G Ratio**
Insulin	**Glucagon**

- Inhibits fat use (lipolysis)
- Increases fat storage
- Inhibits liver glycogen use
- Increases liver glycogen storage
- Inhibits ketogenesis
- Inhibits autophagy

- Activates fat use (lipolysis)
- Inhibits fat storage
- Activates liver glycogen use
- Inhibits liver glycogen storage
- Activates ketogenesis
- Activates autophagy

WHAT MAKES US HUNGRY?

We consider hunger to be a function of whether something is in our stomach. This idea is the driving force behind eating "bulk," like fiber—something to fill you up yet not add to the total calories we consume. However, feeling hunger is more complicated than empty space in our gut. Hunger is partly driven by energy (in calories) provided to our cells—if the cells of our body sense insufficient energy, that can activate a hunger sensation in the brain, which we feel in our stomach. If this weren't the case, every person that received an IV for nourishment would feel like they're starving. This doesn't happen.

In exploring whether energy or dietary bulk is more relevant for hunger, one group of researchers found that if an IV infusion only contained glucose, a person would feel hunger. However, if the infusion also contained some fat, hunger disappeared.[25] In other words, even though the stomachs of both groups were empty, if their cells sensed adequate energy, particularly in the form of fat, the body didn't feel the need to eat, and the person felt content.[26] Energy from a meal conveys greater satiety than bulk—if your cells are fed, they don't care if there's something taking up room in your stomach.

A remarkable example of just how far this can go is the case report of a morbidly obese Scottish man. This fellow began experimenting with fasting and experienced such a rapid health benefit that he simply kept going. Eventually, he did so under medical supervision, ensuring proper hydration and mineral consumption, and ultimately fasted for 382 days![27]

Obviously, fasting is a powerful tool, and as with any "power tools," you need to use it wisely and deliberately. A critical distinction must be made between fasting and starvation. There is no definite time past which fasting becomes harmful, but it can have unintended consequences if taken too far; so much depends on the constitution of the person fasting, how they define "fasting" (what are they drinking, how are they supplementing, etc.), and how they're ensuring essential mineral intake. Also, how a person ends a fast matters greatly. Early studies into prolonged, *multiday* fasting found a potentially lethal consequence called "refeeding syndrome" can develop after fasting ends.[28] Refeeding syndrome happens when blood levels of electrolytes and minerals, such as phosphorous and potassium, become too low. Interestingly, this dangerous shift is caused by insulin suddenly going up too high, too quickly. Thus, just as a body has shifted away from using glucose during a fast, eating too much processed carbohydrate, which will spike glucose and insulin, is the wrong way to end a fast. The calories we eat, when we do eat, have a powerful effect on insulin control, something we'll discuss now.

Circadian Rhythm and the Dawn Phenomenon

Our body has an inherent rhythm and timing to numerous functions that extend well beyond waking and sleeping. Powerful hormones, such as cortisol and growth hormone, ebb and flow throughout the day and night. Insulin naturally follows this rhythm as well; even when we haven't eaten, insulin levels start to climb around 5:30 AM and begin falling within roughly two hours.[29] These rising insulin levels indicate a mild insulin-resistant state, and importantly, this isn't something that only happens when we're sleep deprived—it happens every day, even when we get a full night's sleep. This early morning insulin resistance is known as the "dawn phenomenon" or "dawn effect."

A controlled trial measured the varying insulin levels of people drinking the same amount of glucose during three times of day (morning, afternoon, and evening) and found the insulin response highest in the morning and lowest in the evening.[30] The reason why the body needed more insulin in the morning is a result of hormones that counter insulin's actions. I've mentioned how one of insulin's main effects is to reduce blood glucose by driving it into tissues like our muscles and fat. By contrast, hormones that climb toward the end of our sleep cycle, such as catecholamines, growth hormone, and especially cortisol, act to increase blood glucose. All this forces insulin to work harder to do its job—in other words, creating insulin resistance.

Translated into real food, this means that we need more insulin to control blood glucose when we eat a piece of toast in the morning than we would if we ate that same piece of toast in the evening.[31] With this perspective in mind, what we eat when we wake up may matter more than what we eat any other time of day. No meal has gotten as much attention as breakfast, but usually we hear it isn't to be missed. Considering the insulin resistance we experience every morning, one might be tempted to skip breakfast entirely to fight insulin resistance. What does the research say?

One study randomly assigned 52 obese women who were normally either breakfast eaters or skippers to either eat or skip breakfast for three months.[32] Importantly, both new dietary interventions were lower calorie and *identical* in total calorie number (i.e., even though the breakfast skippers only ate twice daily, they ate the same number of calories as the breakfast eaters). Not surprisingly, everyone lost some weight, but those who ate breakfast during the study lost a bit more. However, a similar study tracked the differences in almost 300 overweight and obese men and women for four months, and those researchers found no difference in weight loss between breakfast skippers and eaters.[33] As you can tell, these similar studies raise more questions than they answer; they don't tell us whether breakfast is good or bad for body fat. To me, the resolution is clear—it all depends on what you're eating for breakfast.

I doubt there's another meal of the day so firmly built on eating some of the worst possible foods. For much of the world, breakfast is often largely a meal of sugar and starch—think juice, cereal, bagels, rice, or toast. As we'll see in the next few pages, if this is your average breakfast, you may as well just skip eating and inject yourself with insulin.

THE CLOCK IN OUR FAT

Interestingly, when it comes to insulin sensitivity, our fat tissue marches to the beat of its own drum. Unlike the body as a whole, which is slightly more insulin resistant in the morning, our fat tissue is *more insulin sensitive* in the morning and least sensitive in the evening.[34] Because insulin inhibits fat burning[35] and promotes fat cell growth,[36] eating an insulin-spiking meal in the morning could add more fat to our frames compared with eating it in the evening.

Carbohydrate Restriction

Once we appreciate that too much insulin is a main driver of insulin resistance, the chain of events suggesting a solution is too obvious: eating fewer carbohydrates = reduced blood glucose = reduced blood insulin = improved insulin sensitivity.[37] With a lowering of insulin comes a sort of resetting (re-sensitizing) of the "insulinostat."

To really appreciate the relevance of the food we eat, we need to establish the effect of each macronutrient on blood insulin. As you can see from the insulinostat chart, dietary protein elicits a mild insulin effect (about two times fasting levels, although this depends on blood glucose levels). Carbohydrate, on the other hand, can elicit a remarkable increase in insulin: more than 10 times above normal, with the height and length of the spike highly variable depending on the carbohydrate and a person's insulin sensitivity. Dietary fat elicits no insulin effect at all.[38] Thus, a diet that limits the insulin spiker (carbohydrates,

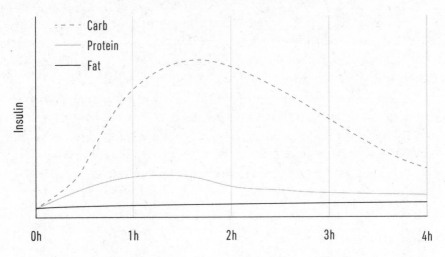

Adapted from Nutall, F.Q. and M.C. Gannon, *Plasma glucose and insulin response to macronutrients in nondiabetic and NIDDM subjects.* Diabetes Care, 1991. 14(9): p. 824-38.

especially refined) and increases the insulin dampeners (protein and fat, especially unrefined) is one that should improve insulin sensitivity. And—as we will see—it does.

There are several relevant topics to discuss with regard to a carbo-hydrate-restricted diet, including the effects on insulin resistance, an overview of ketones, body weight control, and more.

HOW MUCH DOES PROTEIN REALLY INCREASE INSULIN? IT DEPENDS . . .

The overwhelming consensus with dietary protein is that it causes a sig-nificant spike in insulin. However, this is highly dependent on the need for gluconeogenesis (GNG). GNG is the process whereby the liver natu-rally makes glucose for the body when there isn't enough coming from the diet. Due to GNG, eating carbohydrates is unnecessary,[39] though they can still certainly be a pleasant part of the diet. When a person who eats a normal high-carbohydrate diet ingests protein, they experience a robust rise in insulin. However, in a person who eats relatively fewer carbs, they have little or no insulin response to protein.[40] The main rea-son for these different insulin responses is likely based on whether or not GNG is needed. When we eat less glucose, GNG picks up the slack, keeping our blood glucose perfectly normal. Because insulin inhibits GNG so strongly, an insulin spike with eating protein in the context of a low carbohydrate diet would be dangerous—we would deprive the body of its natural and inherent glucose source.

Carbohydrate Intake and Insulin Resistance

Restricting carbohydrates was perhaps the first modern documented intervention to control diabetes and weight, accepted as fact throughout Western Europe in the early and mid-1800s. Why such a paradigm fell out of favor, to be replaced with the current recommendations that those with insulin resistance and type 2 diabetes should avoid fat and eat starches, is puzzling, but the shift in guidelines was dramatic. Within decades (from the early to the mid-1900s), guidelines for diabetes went from encouraging strict avoidance of bread, cereals, sugar, and so forth, while allowing all meats, eggs, cheese, and the like (per *The Practice of Endocrinology* in 1951), to just the opposite—encouraging breads and cereals while discouraging meats, eggs, et cetera (per the American Heart Association and, until recently, the American Diabetes Association). And we responded—we eat relatively less fat now than we ate 50 years ago.[41] This change was supposed to make us healthier, but the explosion of insulin resistance during this time is evidence that our modern dietary shift away from fat in favor of carbohydrates has not yielded the intended results.

Clinical research since the 1990s has provided compelling evidence that carbohydrate restriction prevents or improves insulin resistance. Indeed, when comparing studies that actually change a subject's diet (intervention or clinically based studies) rather than simply asking questions about a subject's diet (questionnaire-based studies), the consensus is overwhelmingly supportive of carbohydrate restriction. Intervention-based studies are far superior because they're able to *definitively* answer questions like, "Which diet is best for improving insulin resistance?" One study that asked this question brought in hundreds of overweight middle-aged men and women. For two years, study subjects were assigned one of three diets: a calorie-restricted, low-fat diet; a calorie-restricted, moderate-fat diet, and a non–calorie-restricted low-carb diet. In addition to causing the greatest weight loss, the unrestricted low-carb diet also helped lower insulin and improve insulin resistance the most.[42]

A different study employed a similar strategy for three months. Overweight men and women were split into either a low-carbohydrate or low-fat diet group; neither group limited calorie intake. While insulin levels dropped by roughly 15% in the low-fat diet group, subjects in the low-carbohydrate diet group saw insulin levels drop by 50%.[43] Moreover, another indicator of insulin resistance (the "HOMA score," discussed more in chapter seventeen) dropped over three times more with the low-carbohydrate diet compared with the low-fat diet.

Yet another study followed its subjects for almost four years while they stuck to a carbohydrate-restricted diet.[44] The thrust of the study was to compare metabolic improvements, including insulin sensitivity, with two interventions—diets containing either 50% or 20% carbohydrate. Not only was the lower carbohydrate diet "significantly superior" at improving health, it ultimately led to almost half of the patients getting off insulin (and almost entirely off any other medications), and the rest substantially reduced daily insulin requirements. A final study worth mentioning is one that put insulin-resistant subjects on a relatively normal diet (~60% carbohydrate) or moderately restricted with carbohydrates (~30%) for three weeks, then switched over to the other diet for another three weeks. Once again, insulin sensitivity increased more with the lower-carbohydrate diet.[45]

I could go on. There are many, many more studies that indicate similar results. Multiple meta-analyses (or statistical analyses that pool the findings from numerous studies), encompassing thousands of patients, unanimously reveal that a carbohydrate-restricted, calorie-unrestricted diet lowers insulin at least as much, and often more, than low-fat, calorie-restricted diets.[46] Indeed, the sum of evidence is so convincing that the American Diabetes Association updated its "Standards of Medical Care in Diabetes" to include the use of low-carbohydrate diets for controlling type 2 diabetes.[47]

Before we move on, it's important to acknowledge that the collective evidence supporting carbohydrate restriction should be viewed in the context of insulin and, thus, should not be considered a call to avoid all carbohydrates. Not all carbohydrates are created equal. Whether they are considered "good" should depend on the degree to which the food increases insulin.

Carbohydrate Quality Versus Quantity

I encourage you to think of carbohydrates as being on a spectrum with regard to their effects on glucose and insulin. It doesn't always matter how many grams of carbohydrate you're eating if the foods you choose have "good" carbs. A useful tool in deciding whether a carbohydrate is "good" or "bad" is by determining its glycemic load, or GL—a number that estimates how much a particular carbohydrate food will raise your blood glucose after you eat it. And, as you know by now, an increase in blood glucose will in turn spike your blood insulin.

It's easy to confuse the GL with the glycemic index (GI). The GI is simply a measure of how *quickly* the carbohydrate is broken down into glucose in the blood. GL, on the other hand, actually determines how *much* carbohydrate is in the food that can become glucose in the blood. Let's take a watermelon, for example. With a GI of 72, watermelon is considered "high GI," but its GL is remarkably low at 2—this means that even though the carbohydrate in the watermelon can rapidly become glucose in the blood (per GI), the actual amount of carbohydrate is low enough to not really matter (per GL). To be clear: The problem with the GI is that it doesn't account for how much potential glucose is in the food you're eating. GL does. Thus, it's possible to consume a diet that has a higher amount of carbohydrates and still potentially prevent or improve insulin resistance if the carbohydrate is low GL. Of course, as a reminder, the underlying utility in understanding the glycemic load is to get an idea of what the food is doing to insulin.

A GL of 20 and above is usually considered "high," 11 to 19 is "moderate," and 10 or below is "low." This convention is fine; just remember, the lower the better. It can be difficult to calculate GL on your own, but there are several online and smartphone app resources that you can use to determine the GL of the foods you're eating.[48] High-GL foods include sugary drinks and candy, white pasta and bread, and French fries and baked potatoes. Whole wheat pasta, brown rice, sweet potatoes, and fruit juices without added sugar generally fall in the moderate range. Some low GL foods are kidney, garbanzo, and black beans; lentils; certain whole-grain breads; and cashews and peanuts.

Fiber-rich vegetables and fruits are good examples of low-GL carbohydrates; a diet high in fiber improves insulin sensitivity.[49] Importantly, for people with insulin resistance, keeping the GL low is significantly more effective at improving health compared with a simple low-fat diet.[50]

Focusing on the GL of foods becomes particularly valuable if your diet is based mostly on plants and plant products (so read closely, vegetarians and vegans). In general, most plant foods are lower in protein and fat and contain mostly carbohydrate (obvious exceptions are "fatty fruits" such as avocado, olives, and coconut). Nevertheless, some plant foods are great sources of dietary fiber that can help control their glycemic effect.

Many of us have heard that plant-based diets are inherently healthier and more effective at preventing disease, though this isn't without debate. Regardless, a plant-based diet isn't necessarily better when it comes to insulin resistance. The simplicity of eating "low-carb" discourages a person from eating any insulin-spiking packaged snacks and treats, such as potato chips. However, such foods could very easily be acceptable on a vegetarian/vegan diet, insofar as they may not contain any animal products.

Again, the GL provides a general and helpful guide (more on this later), though it has its own considerations. What complicates matters is that not everyone responds the same way to carbohydrate foods; GL is an estimated value, but your individual glycemic response may vary.

Glucose Intolerance

We readily embrace the idea that certain people respond poorly to certain foods. We all know people who shun dairy (lactose intolerance) or avoid wheat (gluten intolerance) because of how they feel afterward or what it does to their bodies and health. Is it inconceivable, then, that some of us may respond negatively to dietary glucose?

The idea that some of us have less tolerance to glucose is revealed with a quite simple experiment: people drink a glucose solution and we measure what it does to blood glucose and insulin. Across this group of people, even though fasting glucose levels will be similar, the degree to which the consumed glucose will impact blood glucose can differ widely, including blood glucose levels that rise more than double those seen in others. Importantly, these same people can have equally elevated insulin levels. This is glucose intolerance—where some bodies have to just work harder to move the glucose out of the blood and into the body's cells.

You're likely already suspicious of insulin as a key factor in determining why some people have a stronger response to glucose than others, and you're right. In fact, we know that if the fat cells have become insulin resistant (usually the first cells to "fall," as described earlier in chapter eleven), glucose intolerance will soon follow.[51]

If a person is glucose intolerant, you'd expect them to have a better response to a diet that lowers the dietary glucose—and evidence supports this. In 2007 results were published for a study that sought to rigorously compare the metabolic improvements accompanying four prominent diets—the Atkins diet (~30% carbohydrate), Ornish diet (~60%), LEARN diet (~50%), and Zone diet (~40%). Due to the mix of diets included, the study became known as the "A to Z study." A 2013 follow-up study by these same researchers explored the degree to which insulin sensitivity impacted the response to the diets with the least (Atkins) and most (Ornish) carbohydrates. Interestingly, all subjects lost weight on the lowest-carbohydrate diet, regardless of insulin sensitivity. However, only insulin-sensitive subjects (i.e., those that are the most glucose tolerant), but not insulin-resistant subjects (i.e., those that are the least glucose tolerant), lost weight on the highest-carbohydrate diet.[52]

A GUT FEELING

Differences in gut bacteria could explain how some people are able to readily use carbohydrates and others aren't. That's right—the billions and billions of bacteria in your intestines that help you digest food may be the strongest distinguishing factor that determines how intensely your glucose and insulin respond to a carbohydrate-rich meal. Scientists at the Weizmann Institute found that a person's gut bacteria determined the glycemic load of a food, and that some people had a fairly minor response to things like ice cream, while others had dramatic glycemic responses to common foods like wheat bread.[53]

Saturated and Polyunsaturated Fats

Low-carbohydrate diets are often (not always!) high in animal fat and protein. Many people who avoid animal fat do so out of fear of saturated fat. "The saturated fat will clog your cells and block insulin from working!" is the common cry. There are a few scientific problems with this sentiment.

First, animal fat is never exclusively saturated—it's a broad mix of saturated, monounsaturated, and polyunsaturated. Second, the muscle of insulin-sensitive athletes is just as "fat filled" as the muscle from obese, insulin-resistant people.[54]

However, fat does matter—just not the kind you think. The most likely fat that matters is a type called ceramide,[55] and it's not one you worry about in your diet; it's one you make in your cells. As discussed previously (see page 114), ceramide production is activated by inflammation; once turned on, the cell will turn an innocent saturated fat into ceramide, and the ceramide then makes the cell less sensitive to insulin. Critically, ceramide levels are not increased in the tissues of people who adopt a carbohydrate-restricted, fat-liberal diet.[56] Equally important, saturated fat in the blood is NOT increased in people adhering to a high-fat diet. In one study, the low-carbohydrate group, despite eating three times more saturated fat than the low-fat group, not only had a much greater drop in fasting insulin but also a two to three times greater reduction in saturated fats in the blood![57] In fact, adding saturated fat to a meal (like lard) actually reduces blood fats to lower levels compared with adding unsaturated fats (like olive oil).[58]

One of the dangers with avoiding saturated fat is what we replace it with. Our collective fear of saturated fat has led to an embrace of polyunsaturated fats, derived industrially from seeds. Interestingly, replacing saturated fat (e.g., lard, butter, tallow, etc.) with polyunsaturated fat (e.g., soybean oil, corn oil, rapeseed oil, safflower oil, etc.) may actually do more harm.[59] However, these findings don't apply to all seeds—the polyunsaturated fat (alpha-linolenic acid) from flax seed improves insulin resistance.[60]

The other mechanisms that create insulin resistance, such as oxidative stress and inflammation, are also improved with a diet that is lower in carbohydrates.[61] Thus, carbohydrate restriction addresses several, and the most impactful, of the distinct causes of insulin resistance. However, avoiding insulin-spiking carbohydrates has other effects that help improve insulin sensitivity as well.

Oxidative Stress and Inflammation

I covered how oxidative stress and inflammation can cause insulin resistance in chapter twelve. Here, I want to briefly highlight that while oxidative stress and inflammation are distinct causes of insulin resistance, they're also influenced by the same dietary changes that effectively lower insulin directly—namely, a lower-carbohydrate, high-fat diet. Some of the protective effect against oxidative stress and inflammation could be a result of simply avoiding countless chemicals in seemingly innocent foods; much of the benefit could be from interesting molecules in the blood called "ketones" (described further in a moment). Ample studies have found that ketones elicit potent antioxidant[62] and anti-inflammatory[63] effects.

Having established the efficacy of a carbohydrate-controlled diet in improving insulin resistance, we've really only seen the peak of the mountain of evidence in support of the health benefits of such a diet. Largely because insulin resistance is so prevalent in how multiple chronic diseases develop, countless studies over the past decades have explored the role of low-carbohydrate diets in treating a host of diseases.

Ketogenic Diets

A very low-carb diet is occasionally termed "ketogenic" because of its effects on nutrient metabolism in the body. Specifically, these diets increase ketogenesis—the state when the liver is creating ketones, a nutrient that can be used for energy, from molecules that are produced when the liver breaks down fats (a state called ketosis, as elaborated in the next section). Everyone has ketones; we make them any time insulin is low (or altogether absent, as with type 1 diabetes). With low insulin, the body shifts its energy source to rely heavily on burning fat instead of glucose. This can happen after a period of fasting (e.g., 18–24 hours) or carbohydrate restriction. As fat burning continues, the liver turns some of the fat into ketones, which are essentially a backup fuel for various parts of the body, especially the brain.

Ketones were once considered "metabolic garbage" because scientists were unaware of any role for them. Oh, how the times have changed! Not only are ketones recognized as a viable fuel source for almost every cell, including the brain and muscles, but they're also important signaling molecules that have multiple beneficial effects. Some of the known benefits of ketones include increasing the number of mitochondria in the cell (where fats are broken down),[64] reducing oxidative stress, and controlling inflammation.[65] In the case of some animals, including worms and mice, ketones even extend lifespan, though there is not yet evidence of this in humans.[66] Research from my own lab finds that ketones promote healthy beta-cell and muscle-cell mitochondrial function.[67]

Ketones introduce an interesting option for energy (calorie) accounting in the body. A state of ketosis allows energy to be simply *wasted* from the body, rather than being stored or used. While ketones can be and are used by the body for energy, they are also *removed* from the body through urine and breathing. This is unique to ketones; these "little pieces of energy" allow all the calories to be accounted for while providing a novel "bypass." We are literally passing energetic molecules (i.e., nutrients) from the body in the form of ketones. Each ketone molecule counts for roughly four calories.[68]

Critically, insulin is a powerful inhibitor of ketogenesis—if insulin is high, ketogenesis stops; if insulin is low, ketogenesis occurs. Thus, any diet that keeps insulin consistently low is accurately considered ketogenic.

I consider it necessary to distinguish high-fat diets and ketogenic diets. A high-fat diet, depending on the study, could be one that simply increases fat content without any intervention to lower carbohydrate consumption. Thus, the person on such a vague diet could very well have the same insulin-spiking effect of the typical amount of carbohydrates combined with extra calories from the extra fat. This is decidedly unhealthy. In contrast, a ketogenic diet has replaced carbohydrates with dietary fat. Because dietary fat has practically no effect on insulin, the switch results in a diet that keeps insulin low and, thus, ketones higher than normal.

Ketosis Versus Ketoacidosis

The average diet provides the typical American with blood ketone levels below most conventional methods of detection. This level increases by roughly 10 times when a person adopts a low-carbohydrate diet (blood ketones get to around 1–2 mmol/L). This state, when ketones are increased above "normal" without any effect on blood pH, is referred to as ketosis. But ketones can affect pH if they get too high—when they reach 10 times higher than that found with ketosis (to around 10–20 mmol/L), the blood becomes acidic.

This second 10-fold change is the cutoff between ketosis and ketoacidosis. Most people have negative ideas about ketosis and ketogenic diets because of what they've learned regarding ketones and type 1 diabetes. A person with type 1 diabetes who underdoses insulin will assuredly develop ketoacidosis, which can be life threatening (and not just because of the very high ketones). However, a person with a functioning pancreas will have sufficient insulin production to prevent ketoacidosis, even when fasting.

	Standard Diet	Ketosis	Ketoacidosis
Diet	Frequent eating	Infrequent eating	Untreated type 1 diabetes
	High-carbohydrate	Frequent low-carbohydrate	
Ketones	Insignificant	Meaningful	Dangerous
	Undetectable	0.3 up to ~6 mmol/L	~15+ mmol/L
Blood pH	Normal	Normal	Acidic

Ketone Supplementation

The increasing appreciation for ketones has resulted in the birth of ketone supplements. Because they are so new, understanding the effect of exogenous ketones on insulin control is still in its infancy. However, early evidence is positive. Testing a group of healthy men and women, scientists gave subjects a drink containing ketones, followed soon after by an oral glucose tolerance test (i.e., giving the person a syrupy drink).[69] By measuring blood glucose and insulin levels, the research group found that when fed a ketone drink, the study subjects were able to clear the glucose from the blood more rapidly. Interestingly, and suggestive of the insulin-sensitizing effect of ketones, this occurred without a further elevation in insulin. Participants' levels were similar across the groups; insulin simply worked better.

If you're interested in ketone supplements, just keep in mind that, despite their benefits, drinking ketones is unlikely to help with insulin resistance. In the end, it's the insulin that we care about. Ketones, in the context of insulin resistance, are mostly useful because they're an inverse *indicator* of our insulin levels—they simply tell us how we're doing keeping our insulin in check. For the sake of improving insulin resistance, and all that comes with it, we don't seek high ketones as much as we seek low insulin.

Few people view the food they eat through the lens of insulin resistance; "What will this do to my insulin?" isn't often the question. Overwhelmingly, people ask themselves, "What will this do to my weight?" There is no doubt that the food we eat matters—both how much and what kind. As important as calorie number may be, calorie type is equally important, because it's the type of calorie, whether from fats, proteins, or carbohydrates, that through hormones tells the body what to do with the calories.

Weight Control

At least some of the metabolic benefit of controlling insulin is a result of demonstrable changes in metabolic rate. This is not a recent discovery; two of the greatest scientists in the last century were the first to bring light to insulin's ability to dampen metabolic rate. Elliot P. Joslin and Francis G. Benedict, each now famous for their work in endocrinology and metabolism, respectively, noted in 1912 that metabolic rate in untreated insulin-deficient diabetes was roughly 15% higher compared with similar-body-weight subjects with normal insulin.[70] The same thing can be seen in people with type 2 diabetes treated with insulin: it slows their metabolic rate.[71]

To understand how insulin affects metabolic rate, let's look again at brown fat, or BAT. In the last chapter, we highlighted how BAT helps us burn fat. The metabolic benefits of carbohydrate restriction are not limited to controlling insulin. While insulin inhibits brown fat, ketones activate brown fat.[72] Because of this combination, it's little surprise that an insulin-controlling carbohydrate-restricted diet provides more metabolic "wiggle room" regarding caloric balance than the traditional diet. This could be why people adhering to a *calorie-unrestricted* low-carbohydrate diet can lose more fat than people following the classic *calorie-restricted* low-fat diet,[73] even if potentially eating significantly more calories.[74]

The best example of this is a study that rotated obese and over-weight subjects through four diets that differed in composition of fat and carbohydrates but were identical in calories. Metabolic rate (measured by resting energy expenditure) was the lowest during the lowest-fat diet and increased steadily through the four diets as fat content increased and carbohydrate content decreased. In the end, the metabolic rate of subjects when on the low-carbohydrate, high-fat regimen was roughly 80 calories per day higher than when these same subjects adhered to a low-fat, high-carb diet.[75] More recently, well-controlled studies conducted at both the National Institutes of Health and Harvard University have found the same: when in ketosis, metabolic rate is increased by roughly 100 to 300 calories per day.[76] In the Harvard study, participants were divided into three groups: high carbohydrate (60% carbs, 20% fat), moderate carbohydrate (40% carbs, 40% fat), and low carbohydrate (20% carbs, 60% fat). Additionally, this study used a highly sophisticated technique to measure metabolic rate. Let me elaborate: traditionally, when researchers measure metabolic rate, we either make the person lie down under a space-helmet-like device (indirect calorimetry) or they spend time in a claustrophobia-inducing small room (direct calorimetry); both have obvious problems, since in real life people don't limit their movement like that. The Harvard study, led by Dr. David Ludwig, used a technique called "doubly labeled water," a relatively new and very clever method of determining metabolic rate that allows the subjects to live life as usual by drinking a unique type of "marked" water; researchers measure the rate at which the body uses the water (which is driven by metabolic rate). Metabolic rate changed inversely with carbohydrate consumption; the group eating the highest carbohydrates had the lowest metabolic rate, while the group eating the lowest carbohydrates had the highest metabolic rate. In fact, the group that started with highest fasting insulin levels experienced the greatest increase in metabolic rate with the lowest carbohydrate consumption (this group also had the greatest drop in blood triglycerides and greatest rise in HDL cholesterol).

OTHER BENEFITS OF CONTROLLING CARBOHYDRATES

Earlier, we explored the numerous diseases and disorders that are connected to insulin resistance. If insulin resistance causes these conditions, and controlling insulin is such an effective strategy to address insulin resistance, then an insulin-lowering, carbohydrate-restricted diet should dramatically improve many of those insulin-resistance-connected disorders, right? Researchers have explored this question. Let's take a quick look.

Heart Disease

Blood Cholesterol: Remember that LDL pattern A (larger, more buoyant particles) is less problematic/pathogenic than LDL B (smaller, denser particles). Paradoxically, eating more fat prompts LDL cholesterol to be "more pattern A." One study placed 20 men on either a traditional high-carbohydrate diet or a low-carbohydrate diet for six weeks.[77] Not only did insulin come down significantly, but on average the subjects on the carbohydrate-restricted diet experienced an increase in LDL size. Importantly, even those who were considered pattern B subjects became demonstrably more pattern A due to the increased LDL particle size. A second study conducted an almost identical dietary intervention but followed over 100 subjects for six months[78]; those researchers found similar results.

So, if eating fat and cholesterol, staples in a low-carbohydrate diet, doesn't make LDL more dense, what does? Though rarely explicitly stated, a theme throughout these studies is that eating a diet that keeps insulin low elicits favorable changes in blood lipids; insulin drives an alteration in LDL particles toward small and dense (pattern B). Indeed, the most insulin-resistant individuals have, on average, more than double the amount of small, dense LDL when compared with insulin-sensitive people of similar age and body weight.[79] In summary, a high-fat diet presents a neat paradox—eating more fat has favorable changes in blood lipids.

Blood Pressure: Some traditionalists contend that a high-fat diet promotes higher blood pressure, but the evidence indicates the opposite. In one study, subjects were divided into four diet groups that varied in fat versus carbohydrate intake. In addition to having the greatest drop in triglycerides and the greatest increase in HDL ("good") cholesterol, the high-fat diet group had the largest drop in blood pressure of all the groups—four times greater than the low-fat diet group.[80]

Reproductive Health

PCOS: In a study exploring the role of diet and PCOS, five women with PCOS (who were only mildly overweight) were placed on a low-carbohydrate diet for just 24 weeks.[81] Importantly, the women's amount of free testosterone dropped by almost 25%, which is likely a result of insulin dropping by half (remember that insulin stimulates testosterone production from the ovaries). All the women noted improvements in every self-reported category, including emotional well-being, unwanted body hair, body weight, infertility, and menstruation. Undoubtedly to their great delight, two of the five women, despite repeatedly failed fertility treatments, became pregnant during the course of the study.

Low Testosterone: Men require higher levels of testosterone than women for normal reproductive health. Unfortunately, the staple weight-loss diet we've been following for decades has been hurting that health; putting men on a low-fat diet significantly reduces testosterone.[82] According to the authors of the study, the solution is simple: let men eat more fat.

Neurological Health

Alzheimer's Disease: As we saw in chapter four, several studies in rats have found that a high-sugar diet impairs brain function.[83] Additionally, a study in elderly humans found that those people with the greatest preference for carbohydrates not only ate more carbohydrates, but were the most likely to have the worst neurological symptoms, including the greatest degree of cognitive dysfunction, memory impairment, motor problems, and disengagement.[84]

Humans with Alzheimer's disease or mild cognitive impairment who follow a low-carbohydrate, high-fat diet show improved cognitive function.[85] Interestingly, however, the brain doesn't actually use the fat. When we eat fat as our primary macronutrient, the liver metabolizes more fat than it needs, and the extra fat becomes ketones. In the study just mentioned, the people with the largest increase in ketones had the greatest improvement.

Another study explored this similar dietary effect in 10 subjects, all with varying levels of Alzheimer's-related cognitive decline. (In fact, several had either quit their jobs or were suffering professionally due to the disease.) They ate a low-carb, high-fat diet, fasted 12 hours each night (to increase ketogenesis), and took coconut oil (which is more ketogenic than other fats). All improved their cognitive function and were able to return to work or improve their performance there. The benefits persisted even at a follow-up almost three years later.[86]

In fact, the brain begins shifting to ketone use as ketones become available; this might be evidence that the brain prefers ketones to glucose for fuel. One reason could be that, to a degree, ketone uptake by the brain isn't dependent on insulin, unlike glucose. Thus, if a person is insulin resistant, it's at least possible that their brain has become insulin resistant and takes in less glucose.[87]

Parkinson's Disease: Very few human studies have been conducted on the benefits of a high-fat, low-carbohydrate diet in people with Parkinson's disease. A small study had individuals adopt a ketogenic diet for one month, after which every subject reported "moderate" to "very good" improvements in disease symptoms.[88] A study involving a rat model of Parkinson's disease found that ketones were highly protective of the necessary neurons (e.g., dopamine-producing neurons) because they increased protection against oxidative stress.[89]

Migraine Headaches: The limited evidence that supports the role of ketogenic diets in migraine therapy is almost an afterthought in research. However, it's not new—remarkably, there are published reports from 1928[90] and another, larger report from 1930[91] of improvements in migraine headaches with carb-restricted, high-fat diets.

For example, one study reports that two sisters adopted a carbohydrate-restricted, high-fat diet in an effort to lose weight.[92] Both had reported often suffering from severe migraines. While the sisters adhered to the diet, the migraines resolved; they returned when the sisters stopped. Another revealed that people with insulin resistance who experience migraine headaches (and remember—you may not know you're insulin resistant) could experience a 75% improvement in migraine frequency and severity simply by restricting dietary sugar.[93]

Heartburn

One of the most commonly reported benefits I've heard from people who adopt a carbohydrate-restricted, high-fat diet is the almost immediate reversal of heartburn, the most common symptom of gastroesophageal reflux disease (see chapter seven). Research participants reported experiencing heartburn half as frequently when eating a low-carbohydrate, high-fat diet.[94] Another study detailed five case reports in which all patients who followed this diet had substantial improvements in heartburn.[95] In fact, the study is almost anticlimactic due to the regularity with which it repeats this phrase: "symptoms disappeared within 1 day of starting the low-carbohydrate diet." It may make for a slightly predictable read, but for those who experience heartburn frequently, it's an exciting story!

Skin

Very few studies have attempted to determine the benefit of a carbohydrate-restricted diet for treating skin disorders, but some do reveal positive benefits with acanthosis nigricans,[96] acne,[97] and possibly inflammatory skin disorders, like psoriasis.[98]

> ### Aging
>
> In 2004, a high-profile science manuscript concluded that "endocrine manipulations can slow aging."[99] A diet that keeps insulin low is thus worth exploring. Evidence in insects and rodents is clear: restricting carbohydrates while increasing fat extends lifespan, effectively slowing the aging process,[100] keeping several aspects of the body "young," including maintaining muscle while lowering fat, improving blood lipids, cutting insulin and leptin levels, and improving brain function.[101] Ultimately, these may be among the reasons that families that live the longest tend to be the most insulin sensitive.

The length of this chapter reflects its relevance: when it comes to insulin resistance, the food we eat may matter more than anything else. Our exercise and eating patterns will largely cause or cure insulin resistance. Of course, as powerful as they are, they're also uncomfortable and require meaningful changes. This is likely why they're not more commonly considered and why there will always be a place for easier, if less effective, options.

CHAPTER 16

Conventional Interventions: Drugs and Surgery

B Y NOW, you may be asking, "Can't I just take a pill for this?"
Well, of course you could. Given the prevalence of insulin resistance and its complications, it's perhaps not surprising that countless medical and surgical interventions have sprung up. Prescribing a drug is the most common treatment regimen with insulin resistance. These interventions can improve the *symptoms*. But to varying degrees, they generally fail to address the root causes of insulin resistance.

It is unfortunate, but also understandable, that most physicians' first recommendation is a drug. Before ever interacting with patients, health practitioners will have had countless hours of pharmacology and drug mechanism study, but maybe a handful of hours devoted to lifestyle. What's more, many patients prefer taking a drug to treat their symptoms rather than undertaking the greater effort of changing diet and exercise habits. Yet in most cases, lifestyle changes can completely correct the problem.

Still, it's worth understanding the available medical options. The following table outlines the main drug options, how they work, and the accompanying risks. I've also given each treatment a letter grade based on how well it works compared with its side effects. If diet and exercise alone aren't working for you, you and your doctor may want to discuss one of these treatments.

What is it?	What does it do?
Gliflozin drugs (Farxiga, Jardiance, Invokana, Suglat, Deberza, others in development)	This class of drugs lowers blood glucose by filtering it into the urine. Lowered blood glucose often results in lowering blood insulin. This can lead to weight loss and improved blood pressure.
Thiazolidinedione (glitazone) drugs (Actos, Avandia, Duvie, and Rezulin)	This class of drugs lowers blood glucose by allowing fat cells to divide, thereby pushing more glucose (and fat) into more fat cells. Though these drugs are effective at lowering blood glucose, insulin *levels* may not change very much. Instead, the drugs increase the number of fat cells using that insulin, effectively improving its efficacy.
Sulfonylurea drugs (Glucotrol, Micronase, Amaryl, Glimiprime, and others)	These drugs artificially increase insulin. By increasing insulin, and thereby increasing the existing hyperinsulinemia, the patient reaches normal blood glucose levels. The drugs may also be useful in treating certain neurological conditions.
Metformin (Glucophage)	These drugs directly improve insulin sensitivity at the muscle and liver (and likely other organs), effectively lowering blood glucose and insulin. Used to treat type 2 diabetes and essentially any condition that arises from insulin resistance—especially PCOS and NAFLD
Aspirin	Anti-inflammatory effects improve insulin sensitivity. Used to treat inflammation, reduce risk of insulin resistance, and for type 2 diabetes and atherosclerotic events

How does it work?	What are the downsides?	Grade
All blood glucose is filtered in the kidneys; usually, all the glucose is reabsorbed back into the blood. When blood glucose levels reach an unhealthy level (such as what may accompany diabetes), the kidneys fail to reabsorb all the glucose, instead removing it from the blood and expelling it through the urine. Glifloxin drugs effectively increase this process by blocking the kidneys' ability to move glucose back into the blood.	Increased risk of dehydration due to increased urine production. Glucose in the urine feeds bacteria, increasing risk of UTIs. Limited evidence of increased bladder cancer risk—needs to be confirmed with additional studies.	C
Fat cells are one of just a few cells that require insulin for glucose uptake. Insulin resistance can hinder this effect. By making the body grow more fat cells (hyperplasia), the number of cells that pull glucose from the blood increases.	These drugs almost always increase body fat. From a whole-body perspective, this isn't a great tradeoff—getting fatter isn't an ideal solution to insulin resistance. But the drugs do reduce blood glucose.	B
Once a patient has been diagnosed with overt type 2 diabetes, the insulin resistance has become so severe that the pancreas—though it is still producing plenty of insulin—can't produce enough of it to control blood glucose. These drugs artificially increase insulin production.	Numerous side effects including increased risk of cardiovascular events, abdominal pain, and headaches. Patients often gain a significant amount of body fat.	F
These drugs act specifically to help certain cells be more insulin sensitive. By increasing muscles' insulin sensitivity, they more readily consume glucose in response to insulin, helping drive levels down. In the liver, improved insulin sensitivity reduces the amount of glucose the liver secretes into the blood.	Minor side effects; potential for gastrointestinal irritation, diarrhea, nausea, etc.	A-
Inflammation is a cause of insulin resistance.	High doses (4–10 g per day) have been used in research, and studies into the lowest dose have revealed equivocal results. Main side effects occur in the intestines, including bloating, ulcers, and bleeding.	B+

What is it?	What does it do?
Gastric bypass (also known as Roux-en-Y gastric bypass)	Gastric bypass arguably elicits the greatest improvements in insulin sensitivity among all the bariatric surgeries and the most weight loss, almost immediately curing insulin resistance and type 2 diabetes (~1 week).[3] These rapid improvements precede substantial weight loss, indicating that body fat and insulin resistance aren't always connected.
Adjustable gastric banding	By heavily limiting the amount of food a person can eat at one time, this procedure improves insulin sensitivity.
Sleeve gastrectomy	This is a milder version of a gastric bypass surgery. However, its effects on insulin sensitivity are substantial and very close to those of gastric bypass surgery.[4]

Bariatric Surgeries

Bariatric surgeries have evolved since the 1950s to include several distinct surgical procedures that result in substantial weight loss and improvements in almost all metabolic parameters, including insulin sensitivity. However, the procedure is only performed on individuals who are at a minimum classified as obese, and often obese with complications, such as insulin resistance. All of these procedures reduce stomach size (known as restrictive procedures), but some also further alter intestinal anatomy (malabsorptive procedures).

Before delving in, understand that all bariatric surgeries have frequent side effects, mild to potentially serious, affecting almost half of all patients at some point within six months. Besides the physical side effects, which include severe diarrhea, infections, hernia, vitamin deficiencies, and more, individuals may develop psychological

How does it work?	What are the downsides?
A small pouch is surgically created from the top end of the stomach and a distant portion of the small intestine is attached directly to the pouch, bypassing most of the stomach and the front end of the intestine (duodenum). This results in a state of restrictive eating (the person can only handle a very small amount of food) and malabsorption (the intestines poorly digest and absorb food). Ultimately, the massive food restriction is likely a substantial part of the benefit.	Physical side effects of all bariatric surgeries include severe diarrhea, infections, hernia, vitamin deficiencies, and more. Psychological complications including depression and self-mutilation. About 25% of all patients regain the weight lost in the wake of the surgery, and as the weight returns, the insulin resistance and other disorders return as well.
An adjustable band is placed around the upper portion of the stomach to make the pouch smaller as needed. However, the pouch does not reach the extremely small volume of gastric bypass. Also, the rest of the stomach, beyond the pouch, is still connected, as well as all of the intestine. Thus, all food, once consumed, is digested and absorbed as normal.	Least likely to result in side effects, but also results in the smallest improvements in insulin sensitivity and weight loss.[5] Weight and metabolic problems will likely return once the band is removed.
A significant portion of the stomach (~75%), is removed, and the remaining portion of the stomach is formed into a narrow tube (or sleeve), connecting normally to the intestines. While the sleeve shape reduces volume compared with normal, it's still much larger than the gastric bypass pouch.	Fewer complications than gastric bypass, but more than banding. Interestingly, despite being a simpler procedure than gastric bypass, the changes in body weight and insulin sensitivity are very similar to those seen with gastric bypass. The surgery is irreversible, like gastric bypass—but the benefits can be undone in up to 30% of people if lifestyle doesn't change.[6]

complications like self-mutilation and depression.[1] These surgeries, which involve removing perfectly healthy organs, are a telling sign of our desperation to control metabolic function.

The improvements in body weight and insulin resistance with bariatric procedures are remarkable. Unfortunately, while many of the procedures are irreversible, the weight gain and insulin sensitivity can return. About 25% of all patients regain the weight lost after surgery, and as the weight returns, so do insulin resistance and other disorders. Certain characteristics tend to predict if a person may be more likely to regain, such as depression or evidence of addictive behaviors.[2]

The following table highlights the three most common types of bariatric surgery, how they work, and the accompanying risks. If you are obese and believe you might benefit, you should speak with your doctor about whether you qualify.

CHAPTER 17

The Plan: Putting Research into Action

I N THIS BOOK, I've hoped to bring to light the serious, chronic disorders that can arise from insulin resistance, as well as to arm you with knowledge on the interventions that effectively improve it. However, it won't be worth much without a plan to put this knowledge into action.

As you now understand, the most important changes you can make are lifestyle related. Some are obvious; for example, if you're regularly exposed to cigarette smoke, either make a greater effort to quit or remove yourself from the environment where others are smoking. Some are trickier; indeed, the plan to improve your insulin sensitivity and reduce the risk of the numerous diseases that stem from insulin resistance must revolve around physical activity and, especially, the food you eat. In this chapter, I've translated the findings from all the research I've cited on diet and exercise into guidelines you can follow to make great improvements in your insulin sensitivity. (That said, I always recommend you discuss your plan with your health practitioner, particularly if you have a health condition.)

First, Find Out Where You Are

Before starting any journey, you need to know where you are. If you're planning to make some lifestyle changes to reverse or prevent insulin resistance, first you want to know how insulin resistant you are. So, did you take the Insulin Resistance Quiz (page xviii) at the beginning of the book? If not, go back and take it now. This will give you a general idea of your risk level.

Remember, if you answered "yes" to two or more questions, you're very likely insulin resistant. But don't focus on those symptoms for long. As helpful as it may be to observe and track the symptoms in the quiz, they merely let us know our general insulin sensitivity. For a detailed assessment, you need to measure your insulin levels.

To be frank, there's no easy way do this on your own; there is no at-home, finger-prick test. You need to request a laboratory blood test. And not just any test; every fasting blood test will give you your glucose, but few will reveal your insulin. Thankfully, you have some options. (These options depend heavily on where you live; some countries make this easier than others.)

First, you can request an insulin blood test from your physician. Often the test will be covered by your insurance, but not always (and this is sometimes why the physician may be reluctant). If insurance won't cover the expense, your physician's office can tell you how expensive the test will be, but it is usually under $100 in the United States as of this writing.

If your insurance won't cover the insulin test or you don't want to wait for a clinic visit, you can simply request a test on your own. Numerous companies have sprung up that enable consumers to simply order insulin (and other) tests online. Some examples are walkinlab.com and labtestsonline.org (I'm not affiliated with either). These companies partner with local blood testing services to request the test directly; you go into your local lab, have blood drawn, and the company sends you the results. The test costs around $30 to $60.

Unfortunately, because the focus has been so solidly on glucose for so long, there is not a wide consensus on insulin levels. Ideally, your blood insulin levels should be less than ~6 microunits per milliliter of blood (µU/mL). While ~8–9 µU/mL is the average for men and women, it's not good to be "average" in this case; a person with 8 µU/mL has double the risk of developing type 2 diabetes as a person with 5 µU/mL.[1]

<6 µU/ml	7-17 µU/ml	>18 µU/ml

If you can only get fasting insulin, try to get your blood glucose measured at the same time. The upside of this is being able to figure out your homeostatic model assessment (HOMA) score. This is a helpful little formula that considers both fasting glucose *and* fasting insulin; by covering both sides of the coin, it's more descriptive than insulin alone. The value is determined mathematically by: [Glucose (mg/dL) × Insulin (µU/mL)] / 405 (for the United States) or [Glucose (mmol/L) × Insulin (µU/mL)] / 22.5 (for most other countries). Though there's no consensus yet, a value over 1.5 indicates insulin resistance, and above 3 usually means you're on the borderline of having type 2 diabetes.

Unfortunately, even fasting insulin may have some limitations—there are some people whose fasting insulin may be normal, yet their insulin response to dietary glucose isn't. To do this, working with a healthcare professional or research lab, you drink a small cup of 75 grams of pure glucose and immediately get your blood drawn every 30 minutes for two hours. There are a couple methods to scrutinize insulin,[2] but the simplest is this: 1. If your insulin peaks at 30 minutes and steadily comes down, you're likely insulin sensitive ("Good"); 2. If your insulin peaks at 60 minutes, rather than 30 minutes, be careful—you're probably insulin resistant and your likelihood of getting type 2 diabetes later in life is five times higher than normal ("Caution"); and finally, 3. If your insulin progressively climbs and peaks at 120 minutes, you're most certainly insulin resistant and you're almost 15 times more likely to get type 2 diabetes ("Trouble").[3]

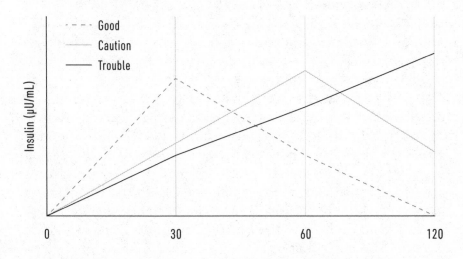

One note on this: if you have type 2 diabetes and you've been prescribed insulin, you can also track your daily insulin dose as a sign of changes. Ideally, you should be checking your blood glucose levels frequently. If, after making some lifestyle choices, your normal insulin dose is resulting in lower than typical blood glucose levels, that dose has become too high—you're more sensitive to insulin. Be warned: Things can change very quickly once you start changing your diet. In fact, in one study of carbohydrate restriction, insulin-treated type 2 diabetes patients had to reduce their insulin dose by half within just a day![4]

If you can't easily measure your insulin, there are a couple of alternatives. One, measure your blood pressure. If you've managed to lower your insulin levels, blood pressure should come down within a few days. Two, measure your ketones. By purchasing a ketone meter, you can get an idea of insulin control, albeit indirectly, insofar as ketones will start to rise as insulin starts to drop. This also may take a few days. You'll recall that a diet that keeps insulin low will also increase ketone production from the liver; this process of ketogenesis is a normal, even healthy, state where the body is using fat at such a high rate that some of the fat is being turned into ketones. Most of the ketones will be used by the body, especially the brain, for energy, but we also expel some in our breath and urine. Because of this, you can measure your ketones in a number of ways. The most accurate—and expensive— is using blood ketone test strips, which are around $1 per strip. The cheapest method is using urine test strips, which cost a few cents each. A final method is a breath ketone analyzer, which falls between both strip methods in expense. All have pros and cons to consider when deciding to take this route.

Many people find it highly motivating to measure ketones to determine how well they're lowering insulin through dietary changes. Though this greatly depends on the person, if blood ketones are around 1 millimole (mM), insulin levels are probably below 10 µU/mL, which is a great insulin level to start with. Unfortunately, using ketones as a marker of insulin changes becomes less useful over time: blood insulin levels may not drop much more, but with ongoing dietary changes, ketones could continue to rise slightly. Until an at-home method of measuring insulin is available, this is the easiest do-it-yourself way to get an idea of your insulin (albeit inversely).

Where You Go Depends on Where You Start

If you're able to get your insulin levels measured, you'll have an idea of where you are now. This gives you an idea of what to do next, which we'll outline later.

If your insulin levels are on the low end (<~6 µU/mL or 41 pmol/L), it's a safe assumption that you're doing quite well, and your insulin sensitivity is strong. You are either already adhering to smart lifestyle choices, or you are young enough to get away with bad choices (for now).

If your insulin levels are moderately elevated (7–17 µU/ml or 48–118 pmol/L), you should start making changes, particularly with the food you eat and how frequently you're eating.

In the event your insulin is high (>18 µU/mL or 125 pmol/L), you need to make changes today. The next time you eat, start making some of the adjustments we'll discuss shortly.

Exercise to Increase Insulin Sensitivity

As we saw in chapter fourteen, using your muscles is crucial in the fight against insulin resistance. If you don't already exercise, it can be tough to know what kind is right for you and how to incorporate it into your life. The best thing you can do right now is not be intimidated by it. We'll explore some helpful ways to start later.

What Kind of Exercise Should I Do?

There is a benefit to any type of exercise, whether aerobic or resistance, though resistance training may offer a greater improvement in insulin sensitivity for the time spent. Nevertheless, before I continue, I feel compelled to state the obvious here: the best exercise to help improve your insulin sensitivity (or achieve any other health outcome) is the one you will actually *do*.

Think of it this way. If you are convinced you should lift weights three times a week to reduce your insulin resistance, but the nearest gym is 30 miles away, you will have a wonderful excuse not to make that drive . . . and you may end up doing nothing. However, if you decide to walk or jog through your neighborhood, even though it may not be as "beneficial" on paper as resistance training, there are far fewer barriers to prevent this from happening (depending on your neighborhood!) and you'll be more likely to do it. So, when committing to an exercise regimen, you will need to determine the genuine limitations in your situation (as opposed to excuses) and act accordingly.

That said, aerobic and resistance exercise are both effective interventions to increase insulin sensitivity, and in an ideal world, your exercise regimen should include both.

To recap: Aerobic exercise is any activity that seeks to more specifically train the cardiovascular and pulmonary systems by increasing the heart and breathing rate. This can be achieved in several ways, including, most commonly, running, cycling/spinning, or swimming.

Resistance training forces a muscle to repeatedly contract or maintain a position against resistance with the intention of developing muscle (and bone) strength. For the novices, some of the exercises described below may be unfamiliar; resistance training has a learning curve. I'd highly recommend becoming familiar with online resources or, if you can afford it, enlisting a trainer to help you become familiar with various exercises and proper movements.

First, the most practical and beneficial method of resistance training is to think "complex." Ideally, resistance training consists of complex exercises that involve complementary sets of muscles (muscles that support the targeted muscles and therefore also get a workout) following realistic movements. A benefit of this method is that you train the muscles to be used in ways that reflect daily life, as opposed to an artificial movement. An example of an artificial movement is the famous biceps curl, where a person raises and lowers a dumbbell by bending their elbow. This movement has almost no real-world equivalent and its only purpose, whether or not the person acknowledges this, is to make a T-shirt fit more tightly around the upper arms.

To fully allow resistance training to produce a stronger, more capable body and improve insulin resistance, separate your lifting exercises into two key motions: pushing and pulling. This deceptively simple scheme allows training to follow natural movement and promotes appropriate and complementary muscle development—muscles that naturally work together become stronger together. For example, strong biceps are useless if your back muscles are weak, because every real motion that involves the biceps (i.e., anytime the elbow closes) involves the back.

Second, if you don't have access to a gym, make do with what you have around your home. Whether it's push-ups and chair squats or lifting water-filled milk jugs and sit-ups, you can fatigue muscles with these "homemade" exercises as well. If your circumstances allow, I'd recommend purchasing a weightlifting bench and a set of dumbbells that match your strength (you'll expand this gear over time).

Third, resistance training is for everyone. Some women avoid resistance training for fear of becoming too bulky; for most women, this simply does not happen. When a man resistance-trains to fatigue on every set, he will get stronger and his muscles will get (potentially dramatically) bigger. When a woman resistance-trains to fatigue, she will get stronger and her muscles will grow a bit and become more defined. Why the difference in size between men and women despite similar relative intensities? It's hormones—the sexes have distinct hormonal cocktails in the blood that dictate the anabolic effects (growth) of the muscle with resistance training. Nevertheless, regardless of size and strength improvements, 60 minutes of resistance exercise in a week can improve insulin resistance more than 60 minutes of aerobic exercise.[5]

DUDE! NO ARM DAY?

Few people have time to devote to the exercises that exclusively work the biceps (front of the arm) and triceps (back of the arm), which is a good thing. Allow these muscles to get worked as they are naturally used, with pushing (triceps) and pulling (biceps) motions. After all, what good is it to have really strong triceps if your shoulders and chest are weak? You won't be any more able to help get yourself out of a chair or off the ground.

Most commonly, people do arm exercises either because they don't know better (forgivable) or they want to show off (unforgivable, but it is easier to show off arms than legs). If you have enough time to focus on the fairly useless (in isolation) muscles of the arm, you'd be better off spending more time on your legs and core.

Remember, friends don't let friends skip leg day.

There are many helpful resources to help you get started on becoming more physically active and training your body to become more insulin sensitive. A very helpful guide is the book *Get Strong* by two fit (and colorful) brothers, Al and Danny Kavadlo, or the You-Tube channel of Jerry Teixeira. To help you get started immediately, I've included a simple exercise plan in Appendix A.

How Often, How Long, and When Should I Exercise?

If you're able, you should engage in physical activity six days per week, reserving one day for a genuine rest to allow the body to recover. Depending on the type of exercise, the daily exercises would need variety to prevent overuse injury and to ensure proper recovery of specific muscles.

I consider 20 minutes to be just enough time capable of eliciting a pronounced benefit. Where time is limited (~20 minutes), intensity of the activity is more important. When possible, 30 to 40 minutes is a good length of time to be certain you fully complete the day's exercise regimen. I personally aim for 40 minutes—anything more, and I feel like I'm mixing my priorities (i.e., spending time with family, etc.).

The time of your exercise session during the day is less important than just getting it done; there is no clear benefit to exercising in the morning versus the afternoon versus the evening. However, people who exercise in the morning usually find fewer excuses and are therefore more consistent. The reality is that fewer things can potentially get in the way of exercising at 6 AM compared with 6 PM.

How Intense Should My Workout Be?

Your exercise intensity may matter more for improving insulin sensitivity than any other variable, including duration.[6] An important caveat: Do not try to do more than you're capable of. When implementing high-intensity training, it is essential to start easier, let your body adapt, and gradually work up to higher intensities.

For aerobic exercise, high-intensity workouts are achieved by simply performing the exercise more vigorously. An ideal way to do this is interval training, where one minute of lower intensity exercise is followed by a minute of maximal intensity, repeated for the desired duration. So, for example, if you choose to run, don't just set your watch for

35 minutes and happily jog away. Rather, keep your eye on your watch to mix intervals of light jogging with periods of heavier running.

For resistance exercise, you can achieve higher intensity by performing every set to failure. In other words, every time you begin an exercise, you continue that exercise, regardless of the number of times it takes (i.e., repetitions), until you can't do any more. Similar to high-intensity aerobic exercise, it's truly exhausting, but it is essential to reaping the maximum insulin benefit. In fact, just a few exercises performed one single time to failure can be enough to improve insulin resistance.[7]

A key benefit for increasing intensity in aerobic and resistance training is that it makes each exercise type more like the other. Just as performing intervals more intensely during aerobic exercise more fully exhausts and strengthens the muscles being used, so, too, does more intense resistance exercise, especially with shorter rests between sets, heavily tax the cardiopulmonary system.

Eating to Keep Insulin Low

Now we've come to what may be the most important lifestyle change you can make. The most scientifically sound diet to improve insulin resistance is one that keeps insulin low. Every aspect of your diet— what you eat, when you eat it—is a means to that end. As you embrace nutritional changes to become more insulin sensitive and help control your health, here are my four vital pillars that provide the foundation of a smart plan:

1. Control carbohydrates.
2. Prioritize protein.
3. Fill with fat.
4. Watch the clock.

As evidence of just how powerful these seemingly simple recommendations are, let me share a recent experience we had in my lab. In working with a local clinic, we had 11 women with type 2 diabetes follow these instructions for 90 days. With no changes in exercise, no counting calories, and, remarkably, without the use of any medications, the type 2 diabetes was gone.[8]

Control Carbohydrates

This is the first and most fundamental principle for rapidly and effectively controlling insulin.

Now, due to inherent metabolic differences among all people, it simply isn't possible to establish a one-size-fits-all strategy. Your ideal composition of macronutrients (that is, the percentage of calories from fat, protein, and carbohydrates) can vary, but no matter what ends up being the right balance for you, carbohydrates will constitute a far smaller part of the diet than is typical in the conventional and ubiquitous "Western diet" (which is typically ~50%–60% carbohydrates). And that's a good thing—we're looking to reverse the trends this diet brought on.

If you answered "yes" to two or more questions from the "Insulin Resistance Quiz" at the beginning of the book (page xviii), you're less tolerant of carbohydrates and, therefore, will need to be more cautious of the type and amount of carbohydrates you eat. If you answered "yes" to only one or none, you'll have more room for carbohydrates in your diet. The reasons for this spread are simply due to how likely it is your body will need make more insulin and keep levels higher for longer to clear the glucose from your blood after eating. Remember that while carbohydrates spark a robust increase in insulin (though there is a broad range; broccoli has little effect, while potato chips have a large effect), protein will have a modest effect, and dietary fat will have none. With this in mind, here are some general macronutrient ranges (percentages of calories from fat, protein, and carbohydrates) that may be helpful as you plan a new nutrition plan to improve or prevent insulin resistance.

- If you answered "yes" to two or more: ~70% of calories from fat, 25% of calories from protein, 5% of calories from carbohydrates
  - Generally less than 50 grams of carbohydrates per day

- If you answered "yes" to one: ~65%–25%–10%
  - Generally less than 75 grams of carbohydrates per day

- If you didn't answer "yes" to any questions (and never want to), you have more freedom: 55%–25%–20% or 55%–30%–15%
  - Generally less than 100 grams of carbohydrates per day (or higher, as warranted by health and physical activity)

Keep in mind that these ranges may require some optimization on your part—these numbers are not meant to be "final." And note that eating less than 50 grams of carbohydrates per day is very likely to be ketogenic in most people. If you're uncomfortable with this and feel strongly that you need more carbohydrates, make every effort to focus on low-GL vegetables and fruits. One thing for all to keep in mind: you don't need to be constantly in ketosis to enjoy the insulin-sensitizing benefits of a carbohydrate-controlled or smart-carb approach.

When it comes to fruits and vegetables, strive to balance carbohydrates and nutrients—choose foods high in nutrients and low in carbohydrates. Be careful to avoid overconsuming high-starch vegetables, such as squashes and potatoes, and high-sugar fruits, like bananas, pineapples, and apples. Here are some good fruits and vegetables (average serving size, 100 g; adapted from www.ruled.me):

Insulin-Friendly Fruits and Vegetables	Fats (g)	Net Carbs (g)	Protein (g)
Cabbage	0	6	2
Cauliflower	0	6	5
Broccoli	1	7	5
Spinach	0	1	3
Romaine Lettuce	1	2	2
Bell Pepper	0	5	1
Green Beans	0	4	2
Onion	0	12	2
Blackberries	1	8	2
Raspberries	1	8	2

Two resources can help you start making insulin-friendly dietary changes. The first is Appendix B of this book, which contains a detailed food list—see pages 209–214. The next is an online database of foods with their respective glycemic loads, which you can find at https://www.health.harvard.edu/diseases-and-conditions/glycemic-index-and-glycemic-load-for-100-foods. Remember the general guidelines for using the glycemic load:

Glycemic Load	Verdict	Examples
<15	Good	Leafy greens like spinach and kale and other nonstarchy vegetables like broccoli, cauliflower, peppers, cucumber, and more; fatty fruits like avocado and olives; eggs; any meat; butter, cheese, and sour cream.
16–30	Be careful	Most alcohol, plain yogurt, whole-fat milk, berries, citrus fruits, most nuts, certain less starchy vegetables like carrots and peas, lentils, and most beans.
>30	Danger	Almost every processed food, juices, breads, crackers, cereals, ice cream, sugary fruits like pineapples and bananas, and so many more.

Along with this general idea of controlling carbohydrates, here are some additional thoughts to consider:

1. Don't be so sweet! An insulin-sensitizing nutrition plan will have very little sugar in it. Mostly this recognizes that sugar is ubiquitous in its many forms. Whether it's "cane sugar," "evaporated cane juice," "high-fructose corn syrup," "brown rice syrup," or others, they're all the same garbage. You can find sugar-free versions of the most common foods in your home, paying particular attention to things like sauces, dressings, ketchup, peanut butter, and so forth. Who wants sugar in these foods anyway, right? You won't taste the difference. When it comes time to actually enjoy a dessert, I encourage you to limit this to only one treat per week or to find a way to make or purchase versions with fewer carbohydrates.

2. Be starch smart! Carbohydrates are an incredibly diverse macronutrient and the more natural the carbohydrate, the better. A general rule to help avoid the worst of the carbohydrates is that if it comes in a bag or a box with a barcode, it's likely a carbohydrate to avoid.

3. Don't drink your carbohydrates. There is a big difference in insulin response when we drink a fruit compared with eating the fruit. When we've removed or altered the fiber in a fruit, we're getting the pure fructose as opposed to fructose with an appropriate amount of fiber. This presence of the natural fruit fiber dramatically reduces the insulin response to the fruit.[9]

4. Where you're able, make an effort to focus on more fermented carbohydrates, like including raw sauerkraut or kimchi (see later) with a meal daily; see below for more about fermented foods. For those who get almost no fermented foods and don't plan on altering their cuisine enough to include them, one easy strategy is to drink apple cider vinegar every day. Whichever is your most carbohydrate-heavy meal of the day, precede that meal with 1 to 2 tablespoons of raw, unfiltered (like Bragg's) apple cider vinegar.

ARTIFICIAL SWEETENERS

Thanks to countless nonnutritive sweeteners, it's possible to enjoy something sweet without spiking glucose and insulin. Be careful with how you buy your sweeteners if you plan on using them for baking or cooking. In general, if the sweetener comes in a powder, it can contain glucose-heavy fillers, such as maltodextrin, defeating the purpose of the sweetener, which is to not spike insulin. Here's a list of sweeteners and how they affect insulin:

Sweetener	Insulin effect alone	Insulin effect with carbohydrates
Sucralose	None	Increased
Aspartame	None	Unclear, possibly increased
Stevia	None	None
Acesulfame-K	Unclear, possible	Unclear, possibly increased
Xylitol	Little	Little
Erythritol	None	None
Other sugar alcohols	Variable, likely	Variable, very likely increased
Monk fruit extract	None	None

THE BENEFITS OF FERMENTED FOODS

Modern conveniences are a blessing in most every way, but, oddly, refrigeration may have yielded unintended consequences on how we digest and ultimately metabolize the foods we eat. Before we could store foods at 39°F to prevent them from going bad, many foods and drinks were, deliberately or not, fermented.

Fermentation involves bacteria digesting sugars (fructose, lactose, glucose, etc.) and producing acids (giving a slightly tart taste), carbon dioxide (giving a drink some bubbles or food some air pockets), and, possibly, alcohol (ranging from trace amounts to high, depending on the nature and length of ferment). The chemical products are interesting, but it's what's lost, not gained, during fermentation that may be particularly relevant in exploring the foods' insulin-sensitizing benefits.

When bacteria are fermenting a food, like a grain, they're not eating the small amounts of fat or protein but rather the starches; bacteria eat glucose. Thus, by eating the starches in the fermenting food, the bacteria help us by lowering the amount of sugars we consume, thereby lowering the effects of the food on blood glucose and insulin. So, we have two pronounced insulin-sensitizing benefits when we consume a fermented food: we consume less starch than the nonfermented version; and we ingest beneficial bacteria that can act as probiotics in our intestines.

Raw apple cider vinegar is a surprisingly effective fermented food. A couple of studies have found that consuming just a tablespoon or so of apple cider vinegar with a starchy meal helps lower the glucose and insulin effect of that meal in insulin-resistant people[10] and may help generally improve glucose control for type 2 diabetes.[11] Also, taking two tablespoons of raw apple cider vinegar in the evening helps control glucose levels the following morning, when glucose levels tend to climb.[12] (This is why I recommend taking two tablespoons of apple cider vinegar in a full glass of water every morning and evening.)

Sourdough, in which natural bacteria allow the bread to rise over time and in the absence of the ubiquitous "fast-acting" yeast, is another remnant of fermented foods in the West. People with insulin resistance who replace normal bread with sourdough bread enjoy a significant lowering of blood glucose and insulin levels.[13] Moreover, sourdough breads have a significantly lower effect on blood glucose compared with normal bread, even when made of the same grains.[14]

If you're in the market for sourdough bread, pay close attention: many are fake. Most "sourdough" breads in your supermarket are actually normal bread with vinegar added to mimic the tart flavor of the real thing. True sourdough bread, rarely sold in supermarkets, will mention "sourdough starter" among the ingredients; it's usually sold in specialty or health food shops. And it's worth it.

Though yogurt has somewhat remained a part of our diet, fermented milk or "sour milk" (note: not the same as spoiled milk!) as an ingredient is now almost entirely absent, though commercial varieties of kefir are beginning to make a comeback. As in sourdough, yogurt bacteria selectively eat the lactose (milk sugar) from the milk, leaving the milk fats and proteins for us. Interestingly, these soured milk products also convey demonstrable protection against insulin resistance: they not only lower the glucose and insulin burden of grains and other foods when consumed with a meal[15] but also improve long-term glucose control.[16]

In contrast to the West, Eastern cuisine has maintained a healthier appreciation for fermented foods. Perhaps the most notable is kimchi, a mix of fermented vegetables. Sure enough, eating kimchi helps lower glucose and insulin levels in people with insulin resistance.[17] Further, this study compared the effects of fresh kimchi against 10-day-old kimchi, suggesting that it wasn't the vegetables that were important, but rather what had happened to them while fermenting. Similar benefits may be seen with fermented ginseng and soybeans.[18]

But eating fermented foods isn't the only way to benefit from the work of beneficial bacteria; probiotics also may do the trick. Probiotics are bacteria you ingest that improve your health, usually in the form of a capsule or powder (if not part of a fermented food). Several lines of evidence support the insulin-sensitizing effects of probiotics; much of this is summed up in a meta-analysis that compiled the findings of 17 randomized trials, concluding that probiotics effectively lower fasting glucose and insulin.[19]

Prioritize Protein

Avoid the temptation to eat too little protein; one concern as people adopt a low-carbohydrate, high-fat diet is that they excessively eschew protein (such as meat or eggs). While certain amino acids (the parts of the dietary protein that flow in the blood) can cause an insulin release, the degree to which this occurs depends heavily on the amount of glucose in the blood, whether the person is ingesting carbohydrate with the protein or has underlying elevated blood glucose (i.e., hyperglycemia). If carbohydrate consumption and blood glucose are low, there will be little or no insulin response to dietary protein. In contrast, if carbohydrate consumption is high and blood glucose is elevated, there will be a substantial insulin response. To optimize muscle and bone growth and recovery from exercise, aim to get 1 to 1.5 grams of protein per kilogram.[20] Critically, if you're older, you need to be on the higher end of this; we become progressively less capable of changing dietary protein into muscle protein as we age.[21]

As stated earlier, eating to control insulin can be achieved in many ways, including via omnivore, vegetarian, and even vegan lifestyles. However, simply due to the relative absence of insulin-spiking starches, eating animal products makes it much easier to control insulin. The foods that contain the most protein, and the least starch and sugar, are animal based.[22]

If you're a vegetarian, you can still follow a smart, insulin-sensitizing nutrition plan. You'll need to search harder to find less starchy and higher-fat menu choices, but they're out there. Avoid the temptation to consume too many seed oils—stick with fruit fats (e.g., from olives, avocados, and coconuts) and, if allowed in your diet, animal fats from nonmeat sources (e.g., dairy, eggs).

If you do eat meat, make an effort to obtain all meat, dairy, and eggs from sources as close to home as possible. Where able, ensure the animals have been pasture raised and allowed to eat their natural diet (e.g., cows eat grass, not grain). While there isn't much evidence to support the idea that free-range meat or eggs are better for health, it's certainly a more ethical and sustainable approach. I suspect you'll be surprised what's available in your area if you take some time to search. The same can be said for those following a plant-based diet; buying locally and avoiding farms that operate "monocropping" can help you be confident that your purchases support a sustainable system. Again, consult Appendix B for a detailed list of insulin-friendly food choices.

Be careful with cured meats, including sausages and especially jerky; these very often include significant amounts of sugar. And don't shy away from fatty meats and fish, including lamb and salmon.

Here's a list of ideal protein sources and their nutritional break-down (based on conventional serving size of 4 oz. or 115 g):

Insulin-Friendly Protein	Fats (g)	Net Carbs (g)	Protein (g)
Ground beef (80/20)	23	0	20
Ribeye steak	25	0	27
Bacon	51	0	13
Pork chop	18	0	30
Chicken thigh	20	0	17
Chicken breast	1	0	26
Salmon	15	0	23
Ground lamb	27	0	19
Large egg	5	0.5	6
Tofu	3	2	7
Tempeh	9	9	15
Pumpkin seeds	42	4	32
Peanut butter	50	14	25

Certain dairy products can be surprisingly high in milk sugars (i.e., lactose). Milk is a perfect example—it's high in all three macronutrients (protein, fat, and carbohydrates), making it an ideal food to help a baby grow (which is why mammals make milk). To focus on good dairy sources that avoid spiking insulin, determine how fermented they've been. As with all other fermented foods, we've allowed bacteria to do some of the work for us—bacteria eat glucose, leaving the fat and protein behind for us to enjoy. Some important examples are cheeses and yogurts. Of course, other ideal dairy sources have just had the protein and carbohydrate removed, such as cream and mayonnaise. Here's a list of good diary choices (average serving size of 100g or ½ cup):

Insulin-Friendly Dairy	Fats (g)	Net Carbs (g)	Protein (g)
Heavy cream	12	0	0
Greek yogurt	1	1	3
Mayonnaise	20	0	0
Half and half	4	1	1
Cottage cheese	1	1	4

Insulin-Friendly Dairy	Fats (g)	Net Carbs (g)	Protein (g)
Cream cheese	9	1	2
Mozzarella	5	1	5
Aged cheddar	9	0	7
Parmesan	7	1	10

GOT MILK? HOLD THE SKIM . . .

Many consider calcium to be the hero of milk, but maybe it's the fat? If you're looking to lose weight, don't shy away from dairy fat. Several studies, including a 12-year follow-up study in men, as well as a prospective study of children, revealed that consumption of whole milk is associated with less risk of being obese or developing obesity compared with consumption of fat-reduced milk.[23] Moreover, very recent analyses suggest that whole-fat dairy reduces the risk of diabetes compared with low-fat dairy.[24]

Fill with Fat

Embrace the insulin-sensitizing value that comes from eating real foods with all their glorious fat. Remember that the fat we eat does not increase insulin and is, thus, a useful food that can nourish your body while not feeding the "beast" (i.e., insulin resistance). In fact, be wary of meals that don't include fat; they won't be as satisfying, and the insulin effect of the meal will very likely be higher than it would otherwise be.

We have a physiological need for dietary fat—it is essential. That doesn't mean all fats are good; the general rule is that if it's a "real" or "natural" fat, it's good, as opposed to fat in processed foods. Also, challenge the dogmatic definition of "healthy fat" as being unsaturated; the more unsaturated a fat, the more readily the fat can be oxidized (and thus harmful—see page 21) and likely to contain unwanted chemicals from being processed. Thus, saturated and monounsaturated fats from animal and fruit sources (i.e., coconut, olive, or avocado) are ideal, and polyunsaturated fats (i.e., soybean oil) should be avoided. Here's a brief primer on dietary fats:

- Saturated fats (good): These include fats from animals (meat and butter/ghee) and coconut oil.
- Monounsaturated fats (good): This is mostly fruit fats (olive and avocado) and certain nuts (like macadamia nut oil)
- Polyunsaturated fats (caution): Polyunsaturated fats from natural sources, like meat and nuts, are fine, mostly because the amounts are so low. This can also include chia and flax seeds, which are rich in one of the three omega-3 fats (i.e., alpha-linolenic acid). Processed seed oils (i.e., soybean oil, corn oil, etc.) and processed foods that contain them have hundreds or thousands of times more polyunsaturated omega-6 fats, making them best avoided.

Another important point about fats and oils is when to eat them in the context of cooking. The more saturated the fat, the more heat it can take; the less saturated the fat (mono- and polyunsaturated), the less heat it can take. In other words, if you're cooking with the oil, use animal fats, like lard or butter, or coconut oil. If you're using the fats/oils as a dressing, the monounsaturated fats are ideal (because they're liquid at room temperature), including olive and avocado oil.

A note on nuts. Like dairy, nuts tend to be higher in all three macronutrients, albeit heavier in fat. Nevertheless, there is a spectrum of carbohydrate content in nuts that is worth noting:

1. Lowest carbohydrate: macadamia nuts, pecans
2. Moderate carbohydrate: This is most nuts, including peanuts, almonds, and walnuts.
3. Highest carbohydrate: pistachios, cashews

Here's a specific list of good ones (based on average serving sizes of 2 oz. or 60 g):

Insulin-Friendly Nuts	Fats (g)	Net Carbs (g)	Protein (g)
Macadamia nuts	43	3	4
Brazil nuts	37	3	8
Pecans	41	3	5
Almonds	28	5	12
Hazelnuts	36	3	9

MICRONUTRIENTS AND VITAMINS

So far in our exploration of diet and insulin resistance, we've focused on the macronutrients—that is, fat, protein, and carbohydrates. There is equivocal evidence on myriad micronutrients, or minerals, vitamins, and other molecules in the diet. The majority of these compounds have no effect on insulin sensitivity, but a handful have been found to have positive results and are worth mentioning. If you feel it would help, consider taking these supplements, though it will in no way compensate for an unhealthy diet; macronutrients matter more than micronutrients.

Magnesium: Magnesium, which is mostly obtained in the diet from leafy greens and nuts/seeds, has generally positive reports with insulin sensitivity. Multiple studies indicate that people with insulin resistance have lower levels of magnesium.[25] In a well-controlled study, subjects receiving 4.5 g of magnesium per day for four weeks were more insulin-sensitive compared with the control group.[26] A somewhat similar study followed subjects with type 2 diabetes[27] for 16 weeks and, again, saw improvements in insulin sensitivity. As evidence of just how beneficial it may be, it appears to even help lower insulin in subjects without diabetes.[28]

Chromium: Chromium is a rarely mentioned mineral whose main dietary sources are green beans, broccoli, nuts, and egg yolks. Within six weeks of taking oral chromium picolinate (400 µg/day), insulin resistance was significantly improved among a group of patients with type 2 diabetes; the improvement was maintained throughout the remaining six weeks of the study.[29] Once the chromium supplementation was ceased, the patients lost the improvements in insulin sensitivity within just a few weeks.

Cysteine: A nonessential amino acid, cysteine can be made in the body if there are sufficient levels of other amino acids (e.g., methionine). Primary food sources are meat, eggs, peppers, garlic, broccoli, and a few others.

Because the data in humans is limited, a rat study is necessarily insightful. Rats were placed on a high-sucrose diet for six weeks and received a low (5.8 grams) or high (20 grams) dose of cysteine. As expected, the high-sucrose diet caused insulin resistance and oxidative stress. However, the high cysteine supplement was sufficient to prevent the increased insulin.[30]

Calcium: When it comes to minerals, many are tempted to claim calcium as the winner for improving insulin sensitivity. However, the results aren't so clear; most of the studies that report a benefit to calcium consumption build the claim based on study subjects consuming more dairy, and the studies that look at calcium alone report no insulin-sensitizing benefit.[31] Dairy, and its various fats, proteins, and carbohydrates, may be helpful, and the calcium may simply be an artifact.

In a group of obese subjects, increasing calcium intake (to 1200 mg/day) by increasing dairy consumption reduced insulin by 18%.[32] However, by placing study subjects on high-dairy diets with or without calcium supplementation, the high-dairy group experienced a remarkable 44% drop in insulin, though the group with calcium had no improvements.[33] In a longer study that tracked overweight subjects for 10 years, the subjects that consumed the most dairy products had the lowest risk of developing insulin resistance and type 2 diabetes.[34]

Vitamin D: We typically think of vitamin D in the context of bone health, but it's a more complicated and beneficial molecule than most think. People who are deficient in vitamin D, in addition to other disorders, will often develop insulin resistance. In fact, the risk of developing insulin resistance is roughly 30% higher than normal.[35] The solution is simple, of course: supplementing 100 µg of vitamin D_3 (4000 IU) per day for just a few months is enough to improve insulin sensitivity back to normal.[36] Other than supplements, great natural sources of vitamin D include fatty fish (like tuna and salmon), egg yolks, and cheese.

Zinc: Zinc is commonly consumed in red meat and, to a lesser degree, poultry. A study in insulin-resistant patients found that those taking 30 mg of zinc daily for six months had significant improvements in glucose and insulin sensitivity compared with the placebo group.[37] However, similar studies reveal no effect.[38]

Watch the Clock!

The most important and simple concept to keep in mind is that having prolonged periods during the day where glucose and insulin are low is a vital step in the right direction. To this end, I recommend adopting a basic strategy of time-restricted eating in some form. I've found a simple and effective method for this.

Fast from food (not water!) for 12 hours every night. Usually, this will take the form of eating dinner around 5–7 PM and not eating again until 5–7 AM or so. Two to three days per week, extend this to an 18-hour fast (e.g., eat dinner at 6 PM and eat your first meal at noon the next day). If your meals are higher in fat and lower in refined carbohydrates, you'll be surprised at how easy this becomes as your body adapts to using fat, including your own body fat, as a fuel, something that can happen as insulin is kept under control. Every two to four weeks, you can even go all the way and fast from food for 24 hours.

Other Tips

As you begin implementing dietary changes that help sensitize your body to insulin and reverse insulin resistance, you will likely find the books *The Art and Science of Low-Carbohydrate Living*; *Eat Rich, Live Long*; or *Protein Power* to be helpful (or any number of books and online sites, such as www.ruled.me). For those who lean more toward vegetarian living, *The Complete Vegetarian Keto Diet Cookbook* and *Ketotarian* will be helpful.

As a general rule, be careful with conventional meal-replacement shakes. This isn't to say you can't use these, but, tragically, drinks marketed for diabetes and weight loss are among the worst due to the grossly misplaced general fear of fat and the surprisingly liberal amounts of refined carbohydrates they contain. Moreover, the fats in most of these drinks are largely seed oils like soybean oil. Thankfully, there are many healthy shakes available nowadays—they just aren't the ones you see conveniently when you're shopping. Just make sure the shakes have *very* little or no sugar or fructose and do not contain seed oils.

Perhaps the greatest challenge with adopting a low-carbohydrate diet is dealing with carbohydrate and sugar cravings. Though the debate rages on around these foods being genuinely addictive,[39] I define food addiction in a simple way:

1. Are you craving the foods?
2. Do you have trouble controlling how much of it you eat?
3. Do you feel guilty when you overindulge?

Nobody is watching a movie at home on a Saturday night craving scrambled eggs; it's chips and ice cream. When you're craving something sweet or salty, try sating the craving with cheese, nuts, or seeds.

And don't forget to check out the detailed food list in Appendix B.

NOT-SO-HELPFUL FRIENDS

Your friends are undoubtedly wonderful, caring people, but be warned—once you commit to eating sweets to only one treat per week, they may suddenly be less than helpful. I've seen many people attempt to make this critical dietary change by reducing sugars, only to have their friends become their most ardent opposition; they seem to tease, if not deliberately sabotage, their friends' efforts to be healthier. It may be human nature—we don't like seeing people make changes we know we should be making, and it's easier to ignore the problem if we're all part of it.

Ideas for Each Meal

BREAKFAST

For reasons discussed earlier, breakfast is arguably the most important meal to change (remember the "dawn phenomenon," page 149). One of the easiest ways to use time-restricted eating to improve insulin sensitivity is to always fast through breakfast.[40] This is a staple of my own insulin-sensitizing strategy, and I've found it's the easiest, most convenient meal to skip.

Changing breakfast is not too difficult because it's usually a meal that is entirely up to you—what you eat won't impact anyone else, unlike lunch and dinner, which you may eat with colleagues or family members (and may limit your choices). Even a breakfast with family can still be selective. After that, here are some ideas of what to eat on mornings when you're not fasting:

1. Bacon and eggs (scrambled in the grease!)

2. Omelets with various veggies (I love adding raw sauerkraut)
3. Egg muffins (blended egg, cream, and cheese baked in small muffin molds)
4. Whole-fat yogurt or cottage cheese with berries
5. Almond milk–berry smoothie

LUNCH

If you eat out, simply find the menu options that provide mostly fat and protein and ensure the carbohydrate is not a refined starch (bread, pasta, potato, etc.). This isn't as hard as it seems—try getting your next hamburger "protein style" or lettuce wrapped. Assuming you "brown-bag it," here are some options:

1. Avocado-tuna salad
2. Cobb salad (with plenty of hardboiled eggs and meat)
3. Protein-style/lettuce-wrapped hamburger (just be careful with the condiments—they're usually high in sugar)
4. Any meat with vegetables
5. Goat cheese salad

I often do simple lunches that are admittedly a bit eclectic (but so simple!), including two or three hard-boiled eggs with salt and pepper, a half cup of olives, a small bag of mixed greens with oil and vinegar, and a stick or two of full-fat cheese.

DINNER

Dinner is where it might get tricky. Depending on your situation and family life, you may find it difficult to change dinner to fit into an insulin-sensitizing diet. The largest barrier is the people you typically eat dinner with—your family (or roommates or significant others) may not want to eat the same way as you, yet you want to (and should) enjoy that social time. Some of this may simply involve you being more selective with what you may already be eating at dinner. Assuming it will be heavier in carbohydrates, you could enjoy having a full glass of water with 2 tablespoons of raw apple cider vinegar before eating. Here are some ideas:

1. Taco salad (skip the shell)
2. Grilled salmon with vegetables
3. Meatballs with vegetable pasta
4. Bacon-wrapped roasted chicken with vegetables
5. Cauliflower mac and cheese
6. Zoodle or vegetable noodle bowls

DESSERT

Dessert? Yes—with sweeteners that don't increase insulin and glucose (e.g., stevia, monk fruit, erythritol, etc.), you can have the sweet without the insulin spike. Nonetheless, this is something that can easily get out of hand and should be considered a rarity (i.e., once per week) rather than a staple. Try:

1. Low-carb ice cream, frozen yogurt, or sorbet (there are more store brands of low-carb ice cream than ever, such as "Rebel"; you could also invest in a home ice cream maker and do it yourself)
2. Low-carb cookies and muffins (like with ice cream, depending on where you live, there are bakeries that specialize in these, such as "Keto Cookie," "Keto Cakes," "Fat Snax," and more)

By now, you've learned enough about how to combat insulin resistance to make a plan and put it into practice. Don't rely on the old way of doing things; there is no need to feel constantly hungry or worry over every calorie. Scrutinizing what and when you eat and the way you exercise to best lower insulin can prevent or even reverse insulin resistance and work to address the countless health problems it causes.

Living with insulin in mind may seem odd, and some of your actions may seem strange to your family and friends, but decades of science are on your side. When it comes to our health and our efforts to live a long and healthy life, it's time to let data, not dogma, dictate our decisions.

IT'S TIME TO TAKE ACTION

STATISTICALLY, you or your loved ones *are* insulin resistant, and if you/they aren't yet, they may be soon; it is *the* most common disorder among adults (and likely even kids) in most countries worldwide. You might not know it, but if you suspect you are insulin resistant or fear you will be, don't wait to make a change. Don't wait until you've gained weight or your blood pressure is climbing or are diagnosed with early-stage Alzheimer's disease, PCOS, erectile dysfunction, diabetes, osteoporosis, or more. If you're concerned about your family history of any of these chronic disorders, you will know you're doing your best to prevent the disease by living a life that keeps insulin low and your body highly insulin sensitive. Reading and understanding a book like this is good, but you need to translate your new knowledge into action.

Do something now:

1. Eat better! Change your breakfast *tomorrow* (and every day thereafter). Either fast through breakfast, or choose to avoid sugars and refined starches and, instead, include fats and proteins from real foods. As you can, change other meals.

2. Get your insulin measured! Most clinics can measure insulin, and online blood test requests are making this easier all the time. If your fasting insulin is above 6 µU/mL, make a change. If your clinician is agreeable, go a step further to measure insulin during an oral glucose tolerance test.

3. Get help! Share some of the relevant studies mentioned in the book with your doctor (he or she may know as little as you did

about this). Go further by including family and friends—teach them what you've learned about how serious the effects of insulin resistance can be, how it develops, and what you can do about it. Remember, statistics suggest they may have insulin resistance (or soon will).

4. Stay informed! As a scientist, I revel in learning more about insulin resistance through my own and others' experiments and published findings. You can easily keep up with the latest published literature by finding me on Twitter (@BenBikmanPhD), Facebook (@BenjaminBikman), and Instagram (@benbikmanphd).

My hope is that by knowing that so many of our chronic disorders share a common origin of insulin resistance, you will feel empowered to make a simple lifestyle change that helps reduce the risk of all of them. Because you *can* do something—your lifestyle, with your individual strengths and weaknesses, genes, and circumstances, is a big part of what got you where you are and, if done right, can get you to where you want to be. Fight the resistance!

ACKNOWLEDGMENTS

THIS BOOK was almost exclusively written between the hours of 4 AM and 6 AM over several years. My inability to sleep more than five hours, and the productivity it creates, is a direct result of my three delightful children (who now all sleep through the night).

My wife, Cheryl, has been very supportive through this process of my "awakening" to the evils of insulin resistance and sharing it with others. When I would talk with her about what I was learning, what once earned me a raised eyebrow now wins an accepting nod—I knew that when she started listening to me, I was really on to something.

My mom and, especially, dad have been highly influential throughout my life. In addition to a slightly off-colored sense of humor, they gave me a love of learning and an appreciation for the decisions required for good health.

My academic ancestry unwittingly placed me on this path. Both Dr. Lynis Dohm and Dr. Scott Summers helped me realize the pathogenic side of insulin and taught me to think more critically and write more effectively.

Faye Atchison, my agent, saw the value in what I know about insulin resistance and helped get a chance to share it in a book. Glenn Yeffeth gave me that chance by agreeing to actually publish it, and the staff at BenBella books, Adrienne Lang, Alicia Kania, Jennifer Canzoneri, Sarah Avinger, James Fraleigh, and Jessika Rieck, helped bring the book to life to share with the world. Specifically, Claire Schulz has been essential in making my writing easy to understand. She is the only person who has read this book more times than me.

My Sample Daily Exercise Plan

HERE IS A STARTER WORKOUT that can be tailored over time as you become more knowledgeable with resistance training and the broad array of exercises. For each exercise, perform two to four sets, going to failure (or very nearly) on each set, usually at around eight to 20 repetitions. If the names of certain exercises are unfamiliar, a simple internet search will reveal the motion. Also, for the sake of simplicity, I've included some "calisthenic" options—exercises that can be performed with only body weight as the resistance.

Monday: Puller leg day

This is a day that will strengthen, among other things, the back of your body, including your lower back, buttocks, and hamstrings.

Weight Training:	Calisthenics:
1. Deadlift	1. Bridge
2. Straight-leg deadlift	2. One-legged body-weight deadlift
3. Reverse lunge	3. Natural hamstring curls

After focusing on the big puller muscles, finish with a focus on calves.

Weight Training:	Calisthenics:
1. Straight leg calf press	1. Standing static calf press
2. Seated calf raise	

Tuesday: Pusher-upper day

This day focuses on the chest and shoulders. Always start with the chest, then proceed to shoulders—all chest exercises require the involvement of the shoulders, and if you start with shoulders, they will be your weak point and your chest will be left "undone."

Weight Training:	Calisthenics:
1. Dumbbell bench press	1. Pseudo planche push-up
2. Dumbbell fly	2. Pseudo planche
3. Push-ups	3. Wall handstand (with or without push-up)
	4. Wide-grip push-up (with or without static hold)

With chest done, finish with the shoulders
1. Standing one-arm dumbbell shoulder press
2. Standing barbell shoulder press
3. Arnold press

Wednesday: Aerobic and Stomach day

This day allows for general recovery, while performing, insofar as possible, a 20-minute high-intensity interval aerobic session (e.g., interval running or cycling) with a series of stomach exercises at the end. One note about the stomach: go slow. Avoid the temptation to speedily complete the motions; rather, perform the motion slowly, contracting the stomach hard throughout the entire motion. Don't relax your stomach at any point—it helps to never let any space come between your lower back and the bench/ground. Also, at peak contraction, exhale powerfully. As usual, go to failure, though it may take ~20 repetitions.

Weight Training/Calisthenics:
1. Knee crunches
2. Leg lifts
3. Heel touches

Remember—go slowly with stomach exercises; form is more important than total repetitions.

Thursday: Pusher leg day

This is an important day, strengthening the muscles that allow you to move around, including running and even simply getting up from the ground or a seated position.

Weight Training:	Calisthenics:
1. Squats	1. Pistol squat (with or without wall assistance)
2. Split squats	2. Box jumps
3. Lunges	3. Single-leg walking lunge
4. Step-ups	4. Standing static calf press

As with puller leg day, finish with some time strengthening your calves.

1. Straight leg calf press
2. Seated calf raise

Friday: Puller-upper day

These exercises target your back, which involves a pulling movement in two ways—pulling with arms above the head, so your hands move toward your shoulders, and pulling with arms in front, so your hands move toward your body.

Weight Training:	Calisthenics:
1. Pull-ups (work up to real pull-ups by using a weight-assisted machine)	1. Any variation of pull-ups (wide grip, narrow grip, archer, etc.; keep chest up throughout)
2. Bent-over barbell row	2. Front lever (start with knees bent and progress toward straight legs)
3. Lat pulldown	
4. One-arm dumbbell row	

Saturday: Aerobic and Stomach day (repeat of Wednesday)

Expanded Food Lists

H ERE IS A FULLER LIST of smart foods to help control insulin, divided
by food category (thanks to www.ruled.me and Insulin IQ for the
resources).

Insulin-Friendly Choices—eat these until you're satiated.

Fats & Oils

Avocado oil	Ghee
Coconut oil	Lard or rendered animal fat
Extra-virgin olive oil	MCT oil
Fish oil	

Dairy (limit your intake if you have sensitivities)

Butter	Cheese (unprocessed)
Cottage cheese	Greek yogurt (full fat)
Cream cheese	Heavy cream

Protein

All meats (beef, lamb, and game)—choose grass-fed if you can	Fish and seafood—choose wild-caught and avoid farmed fish
All poultry (chicken, turkey, and others)—choose pastured if you can	Tofu and tempeh—if you are vegetarian or vegan
Eggs—choose pastured and eat the yolks	

Insulin-Friendly Choices, continued

Vegetables & Fruits (aim for vegetables that grow above ground)

Artichoke hearts	Lemons
Asparagus	Limes
Avocados	Mushrooms
Bamboo shoots	Olives
Bok choy	Onions
Celery	Peppers (bell peppers, jalapeños, etc.)
Cucumber	Radishes
Green leafy vegetables (arugula, chard, lettuce, spinach, etc.)	Watermelon
Jicama	All herbs and spices (basil, cilantro, parsley, rosemary, thyme, etc.)
Leeks	

Fermented Foods

Apple cider vinegar	Sauerkraut
Kimchi	Sourdough bread (look for real sourdough starter in ingredients)
Pickles	

Beverages

Coffee—black or with cream	Unsweetened nut and seed milks (almond, coconut)
Kombucha	Sparkling water—add lemon, lime, or apple cider vinegar
Tea	

Condiments & Sweeteners

Mayonnaise (full fat)	Salad dressings without sugar
Noncaloric sweeteners (erythritol, stevia, monk fruit, xylitol)	

Limit to 2 or fewer servings a day

Nuts, Seeds & Legumes

Almonds	Peanuts
Almond flour and coconut flour	Pecans
Flaxseeds	Pine nuts
Hazelnuts	Pumpkin seeds
Macadamia nuts	Sunflower seeds
Nut butters	Walnuts

Protein

Bacon with no added preservatives or starches	Powdered protein supplements
Fermented soy products	

Vegetables, Fruit & Grains

Barley pearls	Cauliflower
Berries (blackberries, blueberries, cranberries, raspberries, strawberries)	Edamame
Bean sprouts	Eggplant
Broccoli	Kale
Brussels sprouts	Okra
Cabbage	Snap peas

Beverages

Alcoholic beverages (dry wines, clear alcohols, low-carb beer like Michelob Ultra and Select 55)	Whole milk
Flavored fruit drinks with noncaloric sweeteners (Bai, Zevia)	

Condiments & Sweeteners

Greek yogurt dips	Salad dressings containing 2 or fewer carbs or starches
Hummus	Sugar alcohol sweeteners (malitol, sorbitol)

Avoid when possible or eat less than daily

Fats & Oils

Canola oil	Soybean oil
Margarine	Trans fats
Peanut oil	

Dairy (avoid low-fat)

Condensed milk	Skim or low-fat milk
High sugar ice creams	

Protein: Avoid any proteins that are breaded or served with sugary sauces

Vegetables, Fruits & Grains

Apples	Jam, jelly, and preserves
Apricots	Mango
Bananas	Melons
Canned fruits	Oranges
Cherries	Peaches
Dates	Pears
Grapefruit	Plantains
Grapes	Raisins

Beverages

Alcohol (most beer, sweet wines, mixers, and cocktails)	Soda, including diet soda
Fruit juice	Sport drinks (Gatorade)

Condiments & Sweeteners

Agave	Honey
Aspartame	Maple syrup
Corn syrup and high-fructose corn syrup	Sucralose
Fructose	Sugar (white and brown)

RESOURCES

I'VE MENTIONED various books and online resources in *Why We Get Sick* that you may want to read for more information on the issues we've discussed.

Books

- *The Art and Science of Low Carbohydrate Living* by Jeff Volek and Stephen Phinney
- *Good Calories, Bad Calories* by Gary Taubes
- *The Big Fat Surprise* by Nina Teicholz
- *The Diabetes Code* and *The Obesity Code* by Dr. Jason Fung
- *The Alzheimer's Antidote* by Amy Berger
- *Protein Power* by Michael and Mary Dan Eades
- *Always Hungry?* by Dr. David Ludwig
- *The Diabetes Solution* by Dr. Richard Bernstein
- *Eat Rich, Live Long* by Ivor Cummins and Dr. Jeff Gerber
- *The Hungry Brain* by Stephan Guyenet
- *Get Strong* by Al Kavadlo and Danny Kavadlo

Online

- www.ruled.me: Keto diet advice and recipes
- www.dietdoctor.com: Low carb and keto diet advice and recipes
- Body Weight Strength, the YouTube channel of Jerry Teixeira: free online training videos that use only your body for resistance

NOTES

Foreword

1. Jones, D.S., et al., *The burden of disease and the changing task of medicine*. NEJM, 2012. 366: p. 2333-8.
2. Araujo, J., J. Cai, and J. Stevens, *Prevalence of optimal metabolic health in American adults: National Health and Nutrition Examination Survey* 2009-2016. Metab Syndr Relat Disord, 2019. 17(1): p. 46-52.

Introduction

1. Araujo, J., J. Cai, and J. Stevens, *Prevalence of optimal metabolic health in American adults: National Health and Nutrition Examination Survey* 2009-2016. Metab Syndr Relat Disord, 2019. 17(1): p. 46-52.

Chapter 1

1. Menke, A., et al., *Prevalence of and trends in diabetes among adults in the United States, 1988-2012*. JAMA, 2015. **314**(10): p. 1021-9; McClain, A.D., et al., *Adherence to a low-fat vs. low-carbohydrate diet differs by insulin resistance status*. Diabetes Obes Metab, 2013. **15**(1): p. 87-90.
2. Araujo, J., J. Cai, and J. Stevens, *Prevalence of Optimal Metabolic Health in American Adults: National Health and Nutrition Examination Survey 2009-2016*. Metab Syndr Relat Disord, 2019. **17**(1): p. 46-52.
3. Chiarelli, F. and M.L. Marcovecchio, *Insulin resistance and obesity in childhood*. Eur J Endocrinol, 2008. **159 Suppl 1**: p. S67-74.
4. Roglic, G., C. Varghese, and T. Thamarangsi, *Diabetes in South-East Asia: burden, gaps, challenges and ways forward*. WHO South East Asia J Public Health, 2016. **5**(1): p. 1-4.
5. International Diabetes Federation. IDF Diabetes Atlas. 9th ed. https://www.diabetesatlas.org/en/sections/demographic-and-geographic-outline.html. Published 2019. Accessed December 23, 2019.
6. International Diabetes Federation. *4: Diabetes by region*. In: IDF Diabetes Atlas. 9th ed https://www.diabetesatlas.org/upload/resources/2019/IDF_Atlas_9th_Edition_2019.pdf#page=68&zoom=auto. Published 2019. Accessed December 23, 2019.
7. Martin, B.C., et al., *Role of glucose and insulin resistance in development of type 2 diabetes mellitus: results of a 25-year follow-up study*. Lancet, 1992. **340**(8825): p. 925-9; Pories, W.J. and G.L. Dohm, *Diabetes: have we got it all wrong? Hyperinsulinism as the culprit: surgery provides the evidence*. Diabetes Care, 2012. **35**(12): p. 2438-42; Weyer, C., et al., *A high fasting plasma insulin concentration predicts type 2 diabetes independent of insulin*

resistance: evidence for a pathogenic role of relative hyperinsulinemia. Diabetes, 2000. **49**(12): p. 2094-101; Kekalainen, P., et al., *Hyperinsulinemia cluster predicts the development of type 2 diabetes independently of family history of diabetes.* Diabetes Care, 1999. **22**(1): p. 86-92; Crofts, C.A.P., K. Brookler, and G. Henderson, *Can insulin response patterns predict metabolic disease risk in individuals with normal glucose tolerance?* Diabetologia, 2018. **61**(5): p. 1233; DiNicolantonio, J.J., et al., *Postprandial insulin assay as the earliest biomarker for diagnosing pre-diabetes, type 2 diabetes and increased cardiovascular risk.* Open Heart, 2017. **4**(2): p. e000656.

8. Falta, W. and R. Boller [title not available]. Wien Klin Wochenschr, 1949. **61**(14): p. 221; Falta, W., *Insulärer und Insulinresistenter Diabetes.* Klin Wochenschr, 1931. **10**(10): p. 438-443.

Chapter 2

1. Kraft, Joseph R. *Diabetes Epidemic & You.* Bloomington, IN: Trafford Publishing, 2008.

2. Haffner, S.M., et al., *Cardiovascular risk factors in confirmed prediabetic individuals. Does the clock for coronary heart disease start ticking before the onset of clinical diabetes?* JAMA, 1990. **263**(21): p. 2893-8; Despres, J.P., et al., *Risk factors for ischaemic heart disease: is it time to measure insulin?* Eur Heart J, 1996. **17**(10): p. 1453-4; Reaven, G.M., *Insulin resistance and compensatory hyperinsulinemia: role in hypertension, dyslipidemia, and coronary heart disease.* Am Heart J, 1991. **121**(4 Pt 2): p. 1283-8; Pyorala, M., et al., *Hyperinsulinemia predicts coronary heart disease risk in healthy middle-aged men: the 22-year follow-up results of the Helsinki Policemen Study.* Circulation, 1998. **98**(5): p. 398-404; Despres, J.P., et al., *Hyperinsulinemia as an independent risk factor for ischemic heart disease.* N Engl J Med, 1996. **334**(15): p. 952-7.

3. Goff, D.C., Jr., et al., *Insulin sensitivity and the risk of incident hypertension: insights from the Insulin Resistance Atherosclerosis Study.* Diabetes Care, 2003. **26**(3): p. 805-9.

4. DeFronzo, R.A. and E. Ferrannini, *Insulin resistance. A multifaceted syndrome responsible for NIDDM, obesity, hypertension, dyslipidemia, and atherosclerotic cardiovascular disease.* Diabetes Care, 1991. **14**(3): p. 173-94.

5. DiNicolantonio, J.J., J.H. O'Keefe, and S.C. Lucan, *An unsavory truth: sugar, more than salt, predisposes to hypertension and chronic disease.* Am J Cardiol, 2014. **114**(7): p. 1126-8; Stamler, J., A.W. Caggiula, and G.A. Grandits, *Relation of body mass and alcohol, nutrient, fiber, and caffeine intakes to blood pressure in the special intervention and usual care groups in the Multiple Risk Factor Intervention Trial.* Am J Clin Nutr, 1997. **65**(1 Suppl): p. 338S-365S.

6. Chiu, S., et al., *Comparison of the DASH (Dietary Approaches to Stop Hypertension) diet and a higher-fat DASH diet on blood pressure and lipids and lipoproteins: a randomized controlled trial.* Am J Clin Nutr, 2016. **103**(2): p. 341-7.

7. Goodfriend, T.L., B.M. Egan, and D.E. Kelley, *Plasma aldosterone, plasma lipoproteins, obesity and insulin resistance in humans.* Prostaglandins Leukot Essent Fatty Acids, 1999. **60**(5-6): p. 401-5.

8. Steinberg, H.O., et al., *Insulin-mediated skeletal muscle vasodilation is nitric oxide dependent. A novel action of insulin to increase nitric oxide release.* J Clin Invest, 1994. **94**(3): p. 1172-9.

9. Wilson, P.W., et al., *Prediction of coronary heart disease using risk factor categories.* Circulation, 1998. **97**(18): p. 1837-47.

10. Barter, P., et al., *HDL cholesterol, very low levels of LDL cholesterol, and cardiovascular events.* N Engl J Med, 2007. **357**(13): p. 1301-10; Schatz, I.J., et al., *Cholesterol and all-cause mortality in elderly people from the Honolulu Heart Program: a cohort study.* Lancet, 2001. **358**(9279): p. 351-5.

11. Lamarche, B., et al., *Small, dense low-density lipoprotein particles as a predictor of the risk of ischemic heart disease in men. Prospective results from the Quebec Cardiovascular Study.* Circulation, 1997. **95**(1): p. 69-75.

12. Fan, X., et al., *Triglyceride/high-density lipoprotein cholesterol ratio: a surrogate to predict insulin resistance and low-density lipoprotein cholesterol particle size in nondiabetic patients with schizophrenia.* J Clin Psychiatry, 2011. **72**(6): p. 806-12.

13. Selby, J.V., et al., *LDL subclass phenotypes and the insulin resistance syndrome in women.* Circulation, 1993. **88**(2): p. 381-7; Reaven, G.M., et al., *Insulin resistance and hyperinsulinemia in individuals with small, dense low density lipoprotein particles.* J Clin Invest, 1993. **92**(1): p. 141-6.

14. Luirink, I.K., et al., *20-year follow-up of statins in children with familial hypercholesterolemia.* NEJM, 2019. **381**(16): p. 1547-56.

15. Ray, K.K., et al., *Statins and all-cause mortality in high-risk primary prevention: a meta-analysis of 11 randomized controlled trials involving 65,229 participants.* Arch Intern Med, 2010. **170**(12): p. 1024-31.

16. Choi, C.U., et al., *Statins do not decrease small, dense low-density lipoprotein.* Tex Heart Inst J, 2010. **37**(4): p. 421-8.

17. Culver, A.L., et al., *Statin use and risk of diabetes mellitus in postmenopausal women in the Women's Health Initiative.* Arch Intern Med, 2012. **172**(2): p. 144-52.

18. Graham, D.J., et al., *Incidence of hospitalized rhabdomyolysis in patients treated with lipid-lowering drugs.* JAMA, 2004. **292**(21): p. 2585-90; Volek, J.S., et al., *Body composition and hormonal responses to a carbohydrate-restricted diet.* Metabolism, 2002. **51**(7): p. 864-70.

19. Urbano, F., et al., *Impaired glucagon suppression and reduced insulin sensitivity in subjects with prediabetes undergoing atorvastatin therapy.* Eur J Endocrinol, 2019. **181**(6): p. 181-6.

20. Faxon, D.P., et al., *Atherosclerotic Vascular Disease Conference: Executive summary: Atherosclerotic Vascular Disease Conference proceeding for healthcare professionals from a special writing group of the American Heart Association.* Circulation, 2004. **109**(21): p. 2595-604.

21. Steinberg, D. and J.L. Witztum, *Oxidized low-density lipoprotein and atherosclerosis.* Arterioscler Thromb Vasc Biol, 2010. **30**(12): p. 2311-6.

22. Jira, W. and G. Spiteller, *Dramatic increase of linoleic acid peroxidation products by aging, atherosclerosis, and rheumatoid arthritis.* Adv Exp Med Biol, 1999. **469**: p. 479-83.

23. Spiteller, G., *Linoleic acid peroxidation—the dominant lipid peroxidation process in low density lipoprotein—and its relationship to chronic diseases.* Chem Phys Lipids, 1998. **95**(2): p. 105-62.

24. Haffner, S.M., et al., *Insulin-resistant prediabetic subjects have more atherogenic risk factors than insulin-sensitive prediabetic subjects: implications for preventing coronary heart disease during the prediabetic state.* Circulation, 2000. **101**(9): p. 975-80; Festa, A., et al., *Chronic subclinical inflammation as part of the insulin resistance syndrome: the Insulin Resistance Atherosclerosis Study (IRAS).* Circulation, 2000. **102**(1): p. 42-7.

25. Kawashima, S. and M. Yokoyama, *Dysfunction of endothelial nitric oxide synthase and atherosclerosis.* Arterioscler Thromb Vasc Biol, 2004. **24**(6): p. 998-1005.

26. Ridker, P.M., et al., *Comparison of C-reactive protein and low-density lipoprotein cholesterol levels in the prediction of first cardiovascular events.* N Engl J Med, 2002. **347**(20): p. 1557-65; Janoskuti, L., et al., *High levels of C-reactive protein with low total cholesterol concentrations additively predict all-cause mortality in patients with coronary artery disease.* Eur J Clin Invest, 2005. **35**(2): p. 104-11.

27. Krogh-Madsen, R., et al., *Effect of hyperglycemia and hyperinsulinemia on the response of IL-6, TNF-alpha, and FFAs to low-dose endotoxemia in humans.* Am J Physiol Endocrinol Metab, 2004. **286**(5): p. E766-72.

28. Fishel, M.A., et al., *Hyperinsulinemia provokes synchronous increases in central inflammation and beta-amyloid in normal adults.* Arch Neurol, 2005. **62**(10): p. 1539-44.

29. Park, Y.M., et al., *Insulin promotes macrophage foam cell formation: potential implications in diabetes-related atherosclerosis.* Lab Invest, 2012. **92**(8): p. 1171-80.

30. Sakai, Y., et al., *Patients with dilated cardiomyopathy possess insulin resistance independently of cardiac dysfunction or serum tumor necrosis factor-alpha.* Int Heart J, 2006. **47**(6): p. 877-87.

31. Shah, A. and R.P. Shannon, *Insulin resistance in dilated cardiomyopathy.* Rev Cardiovasc Med, 2003. **4 Suppl 6**: p. S50-7; Ouwens, D.M. and M. Diamant, *Myocardial insulin action and the contribution of insulin resistance to the pathogenesis of diabetic cardiomyopathy.* Arch Physiol Biochem, 2007. **113**(2): p. 76-86.

32. Murakami, K., et al., *Insulin resistance in patients with hypertrophic cardiomyopathy.* Circ J, 2004. **68**(7): p. 650-5; Geffner, M.E., T.V. Santulli, Jr., and S.A. Kaplan, *Hypertrophic cardiomyopathy in total lipodystrophy: insulin action in the face of insulin resistance?* J Pediatr, 1987. **110**(1): p. 161.

Chapter 3

1. Bingham, E.M., et al., *The role of insulin in human brain glucose metabolism: an [18]fluorodeoxyglucose positron emission tomography study.* Diabetes, 2002. **51**(12): p. 3384-90.

2. Swanson, R.A. and D.W. Choi, *Glial glycogen stores affect neuronal survival during glucose deprivation in vitro.* J Cereb Blood Flow Metab, 1993. **13**(1): p. 162-9.

3. Porte, D., Jr., D.G. Baskin, and M.W. Schwartz, *Insulin signaling in the central nervous system: a critical role in metabolic homeostasis and disease from C. elegans to humans.* Diabetes, 2005. **54**(5): p. 1264-76.

4. Zhao, W.Q. and D.L. Alkon, *Role of insulin and insulin receptor in learning and memory.* Mol Cell Endocrinol, 2001. **177**(1-2): p. 125-34.

5. Biessels, G.J., et al., *Water maze learning and hippocampal synaptic plasticity in streptozotocin-diabetic rats: effects of insulin treatment.* Brain Res, 1998. **800**(1): p. 125-35.

6. Bourdel-Marchasson, I., et al., *Insulin resistance, diabetes and cognitive function: consequences for preventative strategies.* Diabetes Metab, 2010. **36**(3): p. 173-81.

7. Anthony, K., et al., *Attenuation of insulin-evoked responses in brain networks controlling appetite and reward in insulin resistance: the cerebral basis for impaired control of food intake in metabolic syndrome?* Diabetes, 2006. **55**(11): p. 2986-92.

8. Whitlow, C.T., et al., *Effects of type 2 diabetes on brain structure and cognitive function: African American-Diabetes Heart Study MIND.* Am J Neuroradiol, 2015. **36**(9): p. 1648-53.

9. Kamal, A., et al., *Hyperinsulinemia in rats causes impairment of spatial memory and learning with defects in hippocampal synaptic plasticity by involvement of postsynaptic mechanisms.* Exp Brain Res, 2013. **226**(1): p. 45-51.

10. Querfurth, H.W. and F.M. LaFerla, *Alzheimer's disease.* N Engl J Med, 2010. **362**(4): p. 329-44.

11. Qiu, C., D. De Ronchi, and L. Fratiglioni, *The epidemiology of the dementias: an update.* Curr Opin Psychiatry, 2007. **20**(4): p. 380-5.

12. Accardi, G., et al., *Can Alzheimer disease be a form of type 3 diabetes?* Rejuvenation Res, 2012. **15**(2): p. 217-21.

13. Sadigh-Eteghad, S., M. Talebi, and M. Farhoudi, *Association of apolipoprotein E epsilon 4 allele with sporadic late onset Alzheimer's disease. A meta-analysis.* Neurosciences (Riyadh), 2012. **17**(4): p. 321-6.

14. Kuusisto, J., et al., *Association between features of the insulin resistance syndrome and Alzheimer's disease independently of apolipoprotein E4 phenotype: cross sectional population based study.* BMJ, 1997. **315**(7115): p. 1045-9.

15. Owen, A.M., et al., *Putting brain training to the test.* Nature, 2010. **465**(7299): p. 775-8.

16. Watson, G.S., et al., *Insulin increases CSF Abeta42 levels in normal older adults.* Neurology, 2003. **60**(12): p. 1899-903.

17. Gasparini, L., et al., *Stimulation of beta-amyloid precursor protein trafficking by insulin reduces intraneuronal beta-amyloid and requires mitogen-activated protein kinase signaling.* J Neurosci, 2001. **21**(8): p. 2561-70.

18. Hong, M. and V.M. Lee, *Insulin and insulin-like growth factor-1 regulate tau phosphorylation in cultured human neurons.* J Biol Chem, 1997. **272**(31): p. 19547-53.

19. Schubert, M., et al., *Insulin receptor substrate-2 deficiency impairs brain growth and promotes tau phosphorylation.* J Neurosci, 2003. **23**(18): p. 7084-92.

20. Zolochevska, O., et al., *Postsynaptic proteome of non-demented individuals with Alzheimer's disease neuropathology.* J Alzheimers Dis, 2018. **65**(2): p. 659-82.

21. Owen, O.E., et al., *Brain metabolism during fasting.* J Clin Invest, 1967. **46**(10): p. 1589-95.

22. Contreras, C.M. and A.G. Gutierrez-Garcia, *Cognitive impairment in diabetes and poor glucose utilization in the intracellular neural milieu.* Med Hypotheses, 2017. **104**: p. 160-165; Mosconi, L., et al., *FDG-PET changes in brain glucose metabolism from normal cognition to pathologically verified Alzheimer's disease.* Eur J Nucl Med Mol Imaging, 2009. **36**(5): p. 811-22; Berger, A., *Insulin resistance and reduced brain glucose metabolism in the aetiology of Alzheimer's disease.* J Insulin Resistance, 2016. **1**(1).

23. Kivipelto, M., et al., *Midlife vascular risk factors and Alzheimer's disease in later life: longitudinal, population based study.* BMJ, 2001. **322**(7300): p. 1447-51.

24. Peila, R., et al., *Type 2 diabetes, APOE gene, and the risk for dementia and related pathologies: The Honolulu-Asia Aging Study.* Diabetes, 2002. **51**(4): p. 1256-62.

25. Figlewicz, D.P., et al., *Diabetes causes differential changes in CNS noradrenergic and dopaminergic neurons in the rat: a molecular study.* Brain Res, 1996. **736**(1-2): p. 54-60.

26. Lozovsky, D., C.F. Saller, and I.J. Kopin, *Dopamine receptor binding is increased in diabetic rats.* Science, 1981. **214**(4524): p. 1031-3.

27. Caravaggio, F., et al., *Reduced insulin sensitivity is related to less endogenous dopamine at D2/3 receptors in the ventral striatum of healthy nonobese humans.* Int J Neuropsychopharmacol, 2015. **18**(7): p. pyv014.

28. Pijl, H., *Reduced dopaminergic tone in hypothalamic neural circuits: expression of a "thrifty" genotype underlying the metabolic syndrome?* Eur J Pharmacol, 2003. **480**(1-3): p. 125-31.

29. Henderson, D.C., et al., *Clozapine, diabetes mellitus, weight gain, and lipid abnormalities: A five-year naturalistic study.* Am J Psychiatry, 2000. **157**(6): p. 975-81.

30. Ober, S.K., R. Hudak, and A. Rusterholtz, *Hyperglycemia and olanzapine.* Am J Psychiatry, 1999. **156**(6): p. 970; Sharma, A.M., U. Schorr, and A. Distler, *Insulin resistance in young salt-sensitive normotensive subjects.* Hypertension, 1993. **21**(3): p. 273-9.

31. Aviles-Olmos, I., et al., *Parkinson's disease, insulin resistance and novel agents of neuroprotection.* Brain, 2013. **136**(Pt 2): p. 374-84.

32. Podolsky, S. and N.A. Leopold, *Abnormal glucose tolerance and arginine tolerance tests in Huntington's disease.* Gerontology, 1977. **23**(1): p. 55-63.

33. Schubotz, R., et al., *[Fatty acid patterns and glucose tolerance in Huntington's chorea (author's transl)].* Res Exp Med (Berl), 1976. **167**(3): p. 203-15.

34. Hurlbert, M.S., et al., *Mice transgenic for an expanded CAG repeat in the Huntington's disease gene develop diabetes.* Diabetes, 1999. **48**(3): p. 649-51.

35. Fava, A., et al., *Chronic migraine in women is associated with insulin resistance: a cross-sectional study.* Eur J Neurol, 2014. **21**(2): p. 267-72.

36. Cavestro, C., et al., *Insulin metabolism is altered in migraineurs: a new pathogenic mechanism for migraine?* Headache, 2007. **47**(10): p. 1436-42.

37. Cavestro, C., et al., *Alpha-lipoic acid shows promise to improve migraine in patients with insulin resistance: a 6-month exploratory study.* J Med Food, 2018. **21**(3): p. 269-73.

38. Kim, J.H., et al., *Interictal metabolic changes in episodic migraine: a voxel-based FDG-PET study.* Cephalalgia, 2010. **30**(1): p. 53-61.

39. Grote, C.W. and D.E. Wright, *A Role for insulin in diabetic neuropathy.* Front Neurosci, 2016. **10**: p. 581.

Chapter 4

1. Seethalakshmi, L., M. Menon, and D. Diamond, *The effect of streptozotocin-induced diabetes on the neuroendocrine-male reproductive tract axis of the adult rat.* J Urol, 1987. **138**(1): p. 190-4; Tesone, M., et al., *Ovarian dysfunction in streptozotocin-induced diabetic rats.* Proc Soc Exp Biol Med, 1983. **174**(1): p. 123-30.

2. Pitteloud, N., et al., *Increasing insulin resistance is associated with a decrease in Leydig cell testosterone secretion in men.* J Clin Endocrinol Metab, 2005. **90**(5): p. 2636-41.

3. Dunaif, A., *Insulin resistance and the polycystic ovary syndrome: mechanism and implications for pathogenesis.* Endocr Rev, 1997. **18**(6): p. 774-800.

4. Dimartino-Nardi, J., *Premature adrenarche: findings in prepubertal African-American and Caribbean-Hispanic girls.* Acta Paediatr Suppl, 1999. **88**(433): p. 67-72.

5. Hiden, U., et al., *Insulin and the IGF system in the human placenta of normal and diabetic pregnancies.* J Anat, 2009. **215**(1): p. 60-8.

6. Berlato, C. and W. Doppler, *Selective response to insulin versus insulin-like growth factor-I and -II and up-regulation of insulin receptor splice variant B in the differentiated mouse mammary epithelium.* Endocrinology, 2009. **150**(6): p. 2924-33.

7. Hadden, D.R. and C. McLaughlin, *Normal and abnormal maternal metabolism during pregnancy.* Semin Fetal Neonatal Med, 2009. **14**(2): p. 66-71.

8. Catalano, P.M., et al., *Longitudinal changes in insulin release and insulin resistance in nonobese pregnant women.* Am J Obstet Gynecol, 1991. **165**(6 Pt 1): p. 1667-72.

9. Milner, R.D. and D.J. Hill, *Fetal growth control: the role of insulin and related peptides.* Clin Endocrinol (Oxf), 1984. **21**(4): p. 415-33.

10. Berkowitz, G.S., et al., *Race/ethnicity and other risk factors for gestational diabetes.* Am J Epidemiol, 1992. **135**(9): p. 965-73.

11. Bellamy, L., et al., *Type 2 diabetes mellitus after gestational diabetes: a systematic review and meta-analysis.* Lancet, 2009. **373**(9677): p. 1773-9.

12. Wolf, M., et al., *First trimester insulin resistance and subsequent preeclampsia: a prospective study.* J Clin Endocrinol Metab, 2002. **87**(4): p. 1563-8.

13. Kaaja, R., *Insulin resistance syndrome in preeclampsia.* Semin Reprod Endocrinol, 1998. **16**(1): p. 41-6.

14. Anim-Nyame, N., et al., *Relationship between insulin resistance and tissue blood flow in preeclampsia.* J Hypertens, 2015. **33**(5): p. 1057-63.

15. Koga, K., et al., *Elevated serum soluble vascular endothelial growth factor receptor 1 (sVEGFR-1) levels in women with preeclampsia.* J Clin Endocrinol Metab, 2003. **88**(5): p. 2348-51.

16. Ravelli, A.C., et al., *Obesity at the age of 50 in men and women exposed to famine prenatally.* Am J Clin Nutr, 1999. **70**(5): p. 811-6.

17. Gillman, M.W., et al., *Maternal gestational diabetes, birth weight, and adolescent obesity.* Pediatrics, 2003. **111**(3): p. e221-6.

18. Xiong, X., et al., *Impact of preeclampsia and gestational hypertension on birth weight by gestational age.* Am J Epidemiol, 2002. **155**(3): p. 203-9.

19. Ayyavoo, A., et al., *Pre-pubertal children born post-term have reduced insulin sensitivity and other markers of the metabolic syndrome.* PLoS One, 2013. **8**(7): p. e67966.

20. Phillips, D.I., et al., *Thinness at birth and insulin resistance in adult life.* Diabetologia, 1994. **37**(2): p. 150-4; Byberg, L., et al., *Birth weight and the insulin resistance syndrome: association of low birth weight with truncal obesity and raised plasminogen activator inhibitor-1 but not with abdominal obesity or plasma lipid disturbances.* Diabetologia, 2000. **43**(1): p. 54-60.

21. Friedrichsen, M., et al., *Muscle inflammatory signaling in response to 9 days of physical inactivity in young men with low compared with normal birth weight.* Eur J Endocrinol, 2012. **167**(6): p. 829-38.

22. Li, C., M.S. Johnson, and M.I. Goran, *Effects of low birth weight on insulin resistance syndrome in Caucasian and African-American children.* Diabetes Care, 2001. **24**(12): p. 2035-42.

23. Phillips, D.I., et al., *Elevated plasma cortisol concentrations: a link between low birth weight and the insulin resistance syndrome?* J Clin Endocrinol Metab, 1998. **83**(3): p. 757-60.

24. Yajnik, C.S., et al., *Paternal insulin resistance and fetal growth: problem for the "fetal insulin" and the "fetal origins" hypotheses.* Diabetologia, 2001. **44**(9): p. 1197-8; Knight, B., et al., *Offspring birthweight is not associated with paternal insulin resistance.* Diabetologia, 2006. **49**(11): p. 2675-8.

25. Wannamethee, S.G., et al., *Birthweight of offspring and paternal insulin resistance and paternal diabetes in late adulthood: cross sectional survey.* Diabetologia, 2004. **47**(1): p. 12-8.

26. Marasco, L., C. Marmet, and E. Shell, *Polycystic ovary syndrome: a connection to insufficient milk supply?* J Hum Lact, 2000. **16**(2): p. 143-8.

27. Gunderson, E.P., et al., *Lactation intensity and postpartum maternal glucose tolerance and insulin resistance in women with recent GDM: the SWIFT cohort.* Diabetes Care, 2012. **35**(1): p. 50-6.

28. Velazquez, E.M., et al., *Metformin therapy in polycystic ovary syndrome reduces hyperinsulinemia, insulin resistance, hyperandrogenemia, and systolic blood pressure, while facilitating normal menses and pregnancy.* Metabolism, 1994. **43**(5): p. 647-54.

29. Murakawa, H., et al., *Polycystic ovary syndrome. Insulin resistance and ovulatory responses to clomiphene citrate.* J Reprod Med, 1999. **44**(1): p. 23-7.

30. Mauras, N., et al., *Testosterone deficiency in young men: marked alterations in whole body protein kinetics, strength, and adiposity.* J Clin Endocrinol Metab, 1998. **83**(6): p. 1886-92.

31. Wang, C., et al., *Low testosterone associated with obesity and the metabolic syndrome contributes to sexual dysfunction and cardiovascular disease risk in men with type 2 diabetes.* Diabetes Care, 2011. **34**(7): p. 1669-75.

32. Niskanen, L., et al., *Changes in sex hormone-binding globulin and testosterone during weight loss and weight maintenance in abdominally obese men with the metabolic syndrome.* Diabetes Obes Metab, 2004. **6**(3): p. 208-15.

33. Simon, D., et al., *Interrelation between plasma testosterone and plasma insulin in healthy adult men: the Telecom Study.* Diabetologia, 1992. **35**(2): p. 173-7; Pitteloud, N., et al., *Increasing insulin resistance is associated with a decrease in Leydig cell testosterone secretion in men.* J Clin Endocrinol Metab, 2005. **90**(5): p. 2636-41.

34. Ackerman, G.E., et al., *Aromatization of androstenedione by human adipose tissue stromal cells in monolayer culture.* J Clin Endocrinol Metab, 1981. **53**(2): p. 412-7.

35. Walker, W.H., *Testosterone signaling and the regulation of spermatogenesis.* Spermatogenesis, 2011. **1**(2): p. 116-120.

36. Braun, M., et al., *Epidemiology of erectile dysfunction: results of the "Cologne Male Survey."* Int J Impot Res, 2000. **12**(6): p. 305-11.

37. De Berardis, G., et al., *Identifying patients with type 2 diabetes with a higher likelihood of erectile dysfunction: the role of the interaction between clinical and psychological factors.* J Urol, 2003. **169**(4): p. 1422-8.

38. Yao, F., et al., *Erectile dysfunction may be the first clinical sign of insulin resistance and endothelial dysfunction in young men.* Clin Res Cardiol, 2013. **102**(9): p. 645-51.

39. Sullivan, M.E., et al., *Nitric oxide and penile erection: is erectile dysfunction another manifestation of vascular disease?* Cardiovasc Res, 1999. **43**(3): p. 658-65.

40. Ahima, R.S., et al., *Leptin accelerates the onset of puberty in normal female mice.* J Clin Invest, 1997. **99**(3): p. 391-5.

41. Wehkalampi, K., et al., *Patterns of inheritance of constitutional delay of growth and puberty in families of adolescent girls and boys referred to specialist pediatric care.* J Clin Endocrinol Metab, 2008. **93**(3): p. 723-8.

42. Ellis, B.J., et al., *Quality of early family relationships and individual differences in the timing of pubertal maturation in girls: a longitudinal test of an evolutionary model.* J Pers Soc Psychol, 1999. **77**(2): p. 387-401.

43. Dunger, D.B., M.L. Ahmed, and K.K. Ong, *Effects of obesity on growth and puberty.* Best Pract Res Clin Endocrinol Metab, 2005. **19**(3): p. 375-90.

44. Ismail, A.I., J.M. Tanzer, and J.L. Dingle, *Current trends of sugar consumption in developing societies.* Community Dent Oral Epidemiol, 1997. **25**(6): p. 438-43.

45. Seidell, J.C., *Obesity, insulin resistance and diabetes—a worldwide epidemic.* Br J Nutr, 2000. **83 Suppl 1**: p. S5-8.

46. Lee, J.M., et al., *Weight status in young girls and the onset of puberty.* Pediatrics, 2007. **119**(3): p. e624-30.

47. Soliman, A., V. De Sanctis, and R. Elalaily, *Nutrition and pubertal development.* Indian J Endocrinol Metab, 2014. **18**(Suppl 1): p. S39-47; Ibanez, L., et al., *Metformin treatment to prevent early puberty in girls with precocious pubarche.* J Clin Endocrinol Metab, 2006. **91**(8): p. 2888-91.

48. Preece, M.A., *Puberty in children with intrauterine growth retardation.* Horm Res, 1997. **48 Suppl 1**: p. 30-2; Ibanez, L., et al., *Precocious pubarche, hyperinsulinism, and ovarian hyperandrogenism in girls: relation to reduced fetal growth.* J Clin Endocrinol Metab, 1998. **83**(10): p. 3558-62.

49. Cianfarani, S., D. Germani, and F. Branca, *Low birthweight and adult insulin resistance: the "catch-up growth" hypothesis.* Arch Dis Child Fetal Neonatal Ed, 1999. **81**(1): p. F71-3.

50. Grinspoon, S., et al., *Serum leptin levels in women with anorexia nervosa.* J Clin Endocrinol Metab, 1996. **81**(11): p. 3861-3.

51. Weimann, E., et al., *[Effect of high performance sports on puberty development of female and male gymnasts].* Wien Med Wochenschr, 1998. **148**(10): p. 231-4.

52. Russell, G.F., *Premenarchal anorexia nervosa and its sequelae.* J Psychiatr Res, 1985. **19**(2-3): p. 363-9.

Chapter 5

1. Xu, J., et al., *Deaths: final data for 2007.* Natl Vital Stat Rep, 2010. **58**(19): p. 1-19.

2. Seyfried, T.N., *Cancer as a mitochondrial metabolic disease.* Front Cell Dev Biol, 2015. **3**: p. 43.

3. Kim, J.W. and C.V. Dang, *Cancer's molecular sweet tooth and the Warburg effect.* Cancer Res, 2006. **66**(18): p. 8927-30.

4. Baserga, R., F. Peruzzi, and K. Reiss, *The IGF-1 receptor in cancer biology.* Int J Cancer, 2003. **107**(6): p. 873-7; Peyrat, J.P., et al., *Plasma insulin-like growth factor-1 (IGF-1) concentrations in human breast cancer.* Eur J Cancer, 1993. **29A**(4): p. 492-7; Cohen, P., D.M. Peehl, and R. Rosenfeld, *Insulin-like growth factor 1 in relation to prostate cancer and benign prostatic hyperplasia.* Br J Cancer, 1998. **78**(4): p. 554-6.

5. Tsujimoto, T., H. Kajio, and T. Sugiyama, *Association between hyperinsulinemia and increased risk of cancer death in nonobese and obese people: A population-based observational study.* Int J Cancer, 2017. **141**(1): p. 102-111.

6. Goodwin, P.J., et al., *Fasting insulin and outcome in early-stage breast cancer: results of a prospective cohort study.* J Clin Oncol, 2002. **20**(1): p. 42-51.

7. Papa, V., et al., *Elevated insulin receptor content in human breast cancer.* J Clin Invest, 1990. **86**(5): p. 1503-10.

8. Bodmer, M., et al., *Long-term metformin use is associated with decreased risk of breast cancer.* Diabetes Care, 2010. **33**(6): p. 1304-8.

9. Cleary, M.P. and M.E. Grossmann, *Minireview: Obesity and breast cancer: the estrogen connection.* Endocrinology, 2009. **150**(6): p. 2537-42.

10. Dahle, S.E., et al., *Body size and serum levels of insulin and leptin in relation to the risk of benign prostatic hyperplasia.* J Urol, 2002. **168**(2): p. 599-604.

11. Hsing, A.W., et al., *Insulin resistance and prostate cancer risk.* J Natl Cancer Inst, 2003. **95**(1): p. 67-71.

12. Barnard, R.J., et al., *Prostate cancer: another aspect of the insulin-resistance syndrome?* Obes Rev, 2002. **3**(4): p. 303-8.

13. Albanes, D., et al., *Serum insulin, glucose, indices of insulin resistance, and risk of prostate cancer.* J Natl Cancer Inst, 2009. **101**(18): p. 1272-9.

14. Cox, M.E., et al., *Insulin receptor expression by human prostate cancers.* Prostate, 2009. **69**(1): p. 33-40.

15. Trevisan, M., et al., *Markers of insulin resistance and colorectal cancer mortality.* Cancer Epidemiol Biomarkers Prev, 2001. **10**(9): p. 937-41; Kang, H.W., et al., *Visceral obesity and insulin resistance as risk factors for colorectal adenoma: a cross-sectional, case-control study.* Am J Gastroenterol, 2010. **105**(1): p. 178-87; Colangelo, L.A., et al., *Colorectal cancer mortality and factors related to the insulin resistance syndrome.* Cancer Epidemiol Biomarkers Prev, 2002. **11**(4): p. 385-91.

16. Komninou, D., et al., *Insulin resistance and its contribution to colon carcinogenesis.* Exp Biol Med (Maywood), 2003. **228**(4): p. 396-405; Tran, T.T., et al., *Hyperinsulinemia, but not other factors associated with insulin resistance, acutely enhances colorectal epithelial proliferation in vivo.* Endocrinology, 2006. **147**(4): p. 1830-7.

17. Sukhotnik, I., et al., *Oral insulin enhances intestinal regrowth following massive small bowel resection in rat.* Dig Dis Sci, 2005. **50**(12): p. 2379-85.

18. Katic, M. and C.R. Kahn, *The role of insulin and IGF-1 signaling in longevity.* Cell Mol Life Sci, 2005. **62**(3): p. 320-43.

19. Lee, S.J., C.T. Murphy, and C. Kenyon, *Glucose shortens the life span of* C. elegans *by downregulating DAF-16/FOXO activity and aquaporin gene expression.* Cell Metab, 2009. **10**(5): p. 379-91.

Chapter 6

1. Colman, R.J., et al., *Caloric restriction delays disease onset and mortality in rhesus monkeys.* Science, 2009. **325**(5937): p. 201-4.

2. Mattison, J.A., et al., *Impact of caloric restriction on health and survival in rhesus monkeys from the NIA study.* Nature, 2012. **489**(7415): p. 318-21.

3. Wijsman, C.A., et al., *Familial longevity is marked by enhanced insulin sensitivity.* Aging Cell, 2011. **10**(1): p. 114-21.

4. Bonafe, M., et al., *Polymorphic variants of insulin-like growth factor I (IGF-I) receptor and phosphoinositide 3-kinase genes affect IGF-I plasma levels and human longevity: cues for an evolutionarily conserved mechanism of life span control.* J Clin Endocrinol Metab, 2003. **88**(7): p. 3299-304.

5. Flier, J.S., *Metabolic importance of acanthosis nigricans.* Arch Dermatol, 1985. **121**(2): p. 193-4.

6. Kahana, M., et al., *Skin tags: a cutaneous marker for diabetes mellitus.* Acta Derm Venereol, 1987. **67**(2): p. 175-7.

7. Davidovici, B.B., et al., *Psoriasis and systemic inflammatory diseases: potential mechanistic links between skin disease and co-morbid conditions.* J Invest Dermatol, 2010. **130**(7): p. 1785-96.

8. Pereira, R.R., S.T. Amladi, and P.K. Varthakavi, *A study of the prevalence of diabetes, insulin resistance, lipid abnormalities, and cardiovascular risk factors in patients with chronic plaque psoriasis.* Indian J Dermatol, 2011. **56**(5): p. 520-6; Boehncke, S., et al., *Psoriasis patients show signs of insulin resistance.* Br J Dermatol, 2007. **157**(6): p. 1249-51.

9. Del Prete, M., et al., *Insulin resistance and acne: a new risk factor for men?* Endocrine, 2012. **42**(3): p. 555-60.

10. Frisina, S.T., et al., *Characterization of hearing loss in aged type II diabetics.* Hear Res, 2006. **211**(1-2): p. 103-13.

11. Proctor, B. and C. Proctor, *Metabolic management in Meniere's disease.* Ann Otol Rhinol Laryngol, 1981. **90**(6 Pt 1): p. 615-8.

12. Lavinsky, L., et al., *Hyperinsulinemia and tinnitus: a historical cohort.* Int Tinnitus J, 2004. **10**(1): p. 24-30.

13. Updegraff, W.R., *Impaired carbohydrate metabolism and idiopathic Meniere's disease.* Ear Nose Throat J, 1977. **56**(4): p. 160-3.

14. Srikanthan, P. and A.S. Karlamangla, *Relative muscle mass is inversely associated with insulin resistance and prediabetes. Findings from the third National Health and Nutrition Examination Survey.* J Clin Endocrinol Metab, 2011. **96**(9): p. 2898-903.

15. DeFronzo, R.A., *Lilly lecture 1987. The triumvirate: beta-cell, muscle, liver. A collusion responsible for NIDDM.* Diabetes, 1988. **37**(6): p. 667-87.

16. Goodpaster, B.H., et al., *The loss of skeletal muscle strength, mass, and quality in older adults: the Health, Aging and Body Composition Study.* J Gerontol A Biol Sci Med Sci, 2006. **61**(10): p. 1059-64.

17. Siew, E.D., et al., *Insulin resistance is associated with skeletal muscle protein breakdown in non-diabetic chronic hemodialysis patients.* Kidney Int, 2007. **71**(2): p. 146-52; Park, S.W., et al., *Excessive loss of skeletal muscle mass in older adults with type 2 diabetes.* Diabetes Care, 2009. **32**(11): p. 1993-7; Guillet, C. and Y. Boirie, *Insulin resistance: a contributing factor to age-related muscle mass loss?* Diabetes Metab, 2005. **31 Spec No 2**: p. 5S20-5S26.

18. Pappolla, M.A., et al., *Is insulin resistance the cause of fibromyalgia? A preliminary report.* PLoS One, 2019. **14**(5): p. e0216079.

19. Verhaeghe, J., et al., *The effects of systemic insulin, insulin-like growth factor-I and growth hormone on bone growth and turnover in spontaneously diabetic BB rats.* J Endocrinol, 1992. **134**(3): p. 485-92.

20. Thomas, D.M., et al., *Insulin receptor expression in primary and cultured osteoclast-like cells.* Bone, 1998. **23**(3): p. 181-6.

21. Ferron, M., et al., *Intermittent injections of osteocalcin improve glucose metabolism and prevent type 2 diabetes in mice.* Bone, 2012. **50**(2): p. 568-75.

22. Saleem, U., T.H. Mosley, Jr., and I.J. Kullo, *Serum osteocalcin is associated with measures of insulin resistance, adipokine levels, and the presence of metabolic syndrome.* Arterioscler Thromb Vasc Biol, 2010. **30**(7): p. 1474-8.

23. Skjodt, H., et al., *Vitamin D metabolites regulate osteocalcin synthesis and proliferation of human bone cells in vitro.* J Endocrinol, 1985. **105**(3): p. 391-6.

24. Ronne, M.S., et al., *Bone mass development is sensitive to insulin resistance in adolescent boys.* Bone, 2019. **122**: p. 1-7.

25. Haffner, S.M. and R.L. Bauer, *The association of obesity and glucose and insulin concentrations with bone density in premenopausal and postmenopausal women.* Metabolism, 1993. **42**(6): p. 735-8.

26. Kelsey, J.L., et al., *Risk factors for fractures of the distal forearm and proximal humerus. The Study of Osteoporotic Fractures Research Group.* Am J Epidemiol, 1992. **135**(5): p. 477-89.

27. Erbagci, A.B., et al., *Serum prolidase activity as a marker of osteoporosis in type 2 diabetes mellitus.* Clin Biochem, 2002. **35**(4): p. 263-8; Krakauer, J.C., et al., *Bone loss and bone turnover in diabetes.* Diabetes, 1995. **44**(7): p. 775-82; Isaia, G.C., et al., *Bone metabolism in type 2 diabetes mellitus.* Acta Diabetol, 1999. **36**(1-2): p. 35-8.

28. Thrailkill, K.M., et al., *Is insulin an anabolic agent in bone? Dissecting the diabetic bone for clues.* Am J Physiol Endocrinol Metab, 2005. **289**(5): p. E735-45.

29. Faulhaber, G.A., et al., *Low bone mineral density is associated with insulin resistance in bone marrow transplant subjects.* Bone Marrow Transplant, 2009. **43**(12): p. 953-7.

30. Silveri, F., et al., *Serum levels of insulin in overweight patients with osteoarthritis of the knee.* J Rheumatol, 1994. **21**(10): p. 1899-902.

31. Mobasheri, A., et al., *Glucose transport and metabolism in chondrocytes: a key to understanding chondrogenesis, skeletal development and cartilage degradation in osteoarthritis.* Histol Histopathol, 2002. **17**(4): p. 1239-67.

32. Qiao, L., Li, Y., Sun, S., *Insulin exacerbates inflammation in fibroblast-like synoviocytes.* Inflammation, 2020. doi: 10.1007/s10753-020-01178-0.

33. Svenson, K.L., et al., *Impaired glucose handling in active rheumatoid arthritis: relationship to peripheral insulin resistance.* Metabolism, 1988. **37**(2): p. 125-30.

34. Clegg, D.O., et al., *Glucosamine, chondroitin sulfate, and the two in combination for painful knee osteoarthritis.* N Engl J Med, 2006. **354**(8): p. 795-808.

35. Pham, T., et al., *Oral glucosamine in doses used to treat osteoarthritis worsens insulin resistance.* Am J Med Sci, 2007. **333**(6): p. 333-9.

36. Vuorinen-Markkola, H. and H. Yki-Jarvinen, *Hyperuricemia and insulin resistance.* J Clin Endocrinol Metab, 1994. **78**(1): p. 25-9.

Chapter 7

1. Locke, G.R., 3rd, et al., *Prevalence and clinical spectrum of gastroesophageal reflux: a population-based study in Olmsted County, Minnesota.* Gastroenterology, 1997. **112**(5): p. 1448-56.

2. Chung, S.J., et al., *Metabolic syndrome and visceral obesity as risk factors for reflux oesophagitis: a cross-sectional case-control study of 7078 Koreans undergoing health check-ups.* Gut, 2008. **57**(10): p. 1360-5.

3. Hsu, C.S., et al., *Increasing insulin resistance is associated with increased severity and prevalence of gastro-oesophageal reflux disease.* Aliment Pharmacol Ther, 2011. **34**(8): p. 994-1004.

4. Duggan, C., et al., *Association between markers of obesity and progression from Barrett's esophagus to esophageal adenocarcinoma.* Clin Gastroenterol Hepatol, 2013. **11**(8): p. 934-43.

5. Cameron, A.J., et al., *Adenocarcinoma of the esophagogastric junction and Barrett's esophagus.* Gastroenterology, 1995. **109**(5): p. 1541-6.

6. Guy, R.J., et al., *Diabetic gastroparesis from autonomic neuropathy: surgical considerations and changes in vagus nerve morphology.* J Neurol Neurosurg Psychiatry, 1984. **47**(7): p. 686-91; Annese, V., et al., *Gastrointestinal motor dysfunction, symptoms, and neuropathy in noninsulin-dependent (type 2) diabetes mellitus.* J Clin Gastroenterol, 1999. **29**(2): p. 171-7.

7. Eliasson, B., et al., *Hyperinsulinaemia impairs gastrointestinal motility and slows carbohydrate absorption.* Diabetologia, 1995. **38**(1): p. 79-85.

8. Playford, R.J., et al., *Use of the alpha glucosidase inhibitor acarbose in patients with 'Middleton syndrome': normal gastric anatomy but with accelerated gastric emptying causing postprandial reactive hypoglycemia and diarrhea.* Can J Gastroenterol, 2013. **27**(7): p. 403-4.

9. Johnsson, K.M., et al., *Urinary tract infections in patients with diabetes treated with dapagliflozin.* J Diabetes Complications, 2013. **27**(5): p. 473-8.

10. Kraegen, E.W., et al., *Development of muscle insulin resistance after liver insulin resistance in high-fat-fed rats.* Diabetes, 1991. **40**(11): p. 1397-403.

11. Li, S., M.S. Brown, and J.L. Goldstein, *Bifurcation of insulin signaling pathway in rat liver: mTORC1 required for stimulation of lipogenesis, but not inhibition of gluconeogenesis.* Proc Natl Acad Sci U S A, 2010. **107**(8): p. 3441-6.

12. Choi, S.H. and H.N. Ginsberg, *Increased very low density lipoprotein (VLDL) secretion, hepatic steatosis, and insulin resistance.* Trends Endocrinol Metab, 2011. **22**(9): p. 353-63.

13. Ruhl, C.E. and J.E. Everhart, *Fatty liver indices in the multiethnic United States National Health and Nutrition Examination Survey.* Aliment Pharmacol Ther, 2015. **41**(1): p. 65-76.

14. Paschos, P. and K. Paletas, *Non alcoholic fatty liver disease and metabolic syndrome.* Hippokratia, 2009. **13**(1): p. 9-19.

15. Le, K.A., et al., *Fructose overconsumption causes dyslipidemia and ectopic lipid deposition in healthy subjects with and without a family history of type 2 diabetes.* Am J Clin Nutr, 2009. **89**(6): p. 1760-5.

16. Stanhope, K.L., et al., *Consuming fructose-sweetened, not glucose-sweetened, beverages increases visceral adiposity and lipids and decreases insulin sensitivity in overweight/obese humans.* J Clin Invest, 2009. **119**(5): p. 1322-34.

17. Vos, M.B., et al., *Dietary fructose consumption among US children and adults: the Third National Health and Nutrition Examination Survey.* Medscape J Med, 2008. **10**(7): p. 160.

18. Wojcicki, J.M. and M.B. Heyman, *Reducing childhood obesity by eliminating 100% fruit juice.* Am J Public Health, 2012. **102**(9): p. 1630-3.

19. Bray, G.A., S.J. Nielsen, and B.M. Popkin, *Consumption of high-fructose corn syrup in beverages may play a role in the epidemic of obesity.* Am J Clin Nutr, 2004. **79**(4): p. 537-43.

20. Yuan, J., et al., *Fatty Liver Disease Caused by High-Alcohol-Producing Klebsiella pneumoniae.* Cell Metab, 2019. **30**(4): p. 675-88 e7.

21. Marchesini, G., et al., *Association of nonalcoholic fatty liver disease with insulin resistance.* Am J Med, 1999. **107**(5): p. 450-5.

22. Fabbrini, E. and F. Magkos, *Hepatic steatosis as a marker of metabolic dysfunction.* Nutrients, 2015. **7**(6): p. 4995-5019.

23. Sheth, S.G., F.D. Gordon, and S. Chopra, *Nonalcoholic steatohepatitis.* Ann Intern Med, 1997. **126**(2): p. 137-45.

24. El-Serag, H.B., *Hepatocellular carcinoma: recent trends in the United States.* Gastroenterology, 2004. **127**(5 Suppl 1): p. S27-34.

25. Fartoux, L., et al., *Insulin resistance is a cause of steatosis and fibrosis progression in chronic hepatitis C.* Gut, 2005. **54**(7): p. 1003-8.

26. D'Souza, R., C.A. Sabin, and G.R. Foster, *Insulin resistance plays a significant role in liver fibrosis in chronic hepatitis C and in the response to antiviral therapy.* Am J Gastroenterol, 2005. **100**(7): p. 1509-15.

27. Tsai, C.J., et al., *Macronutrients and insulin resistance in cholesterol gallstone disease.* Am J Gastroenterol, 2008. **103**(11): p. 2932-9; Mendez-Sanchez, N., et al., *Metabolic syndrome as a risk factor for gallstone disease.* World J Gastroenterol, 2005. **11**(11): p. 1653-7.

28. Dubrac, S., et al., *Insulin injections enhance cholesterol gallstone incidence by changing the biliary cholesterol saturation index and apo A-I concentration in hamsters fed a lithogenic diet.* J Hepatol, 2001. **35**(5): p. 550-7.

29. Biddinger, S.B., et al., *Hepatic insulin resistance directly promotes formation of cholesterol gallstones.* Nat Med, 2008. **14**(7): p. 778-82.

30. Festi, D., et al., *Gallbladder motility and gallstone formation in obese patients following very low calorie diets. Use it (fat) to lose it (well).* Int J Obes Relat Metab Disord, 1998. **22**(6): p. 592-600.

31. Nakeeb, A., et al., *Insulin resistance causes human gallbladder dysmotility.* J Gastrointest Surg, 2006. **10**(7): p. 940-8; discussion 948-9.

32. Gielkens, H.A., et al., *Effect of insulin on basal and cholecystokinin-stimulated gallbladder motility in humans.* J Hepatol, 1998. **28**(4): p. 595-602.

33. Maringhini, A., et al., *Biliary sludge and gallstones in pregnancy: incidence, risk factors, and natural history.* Ann Intern Med, 1993. **119**(2): p. 116-20.

34. Maringhini, A., et al., *Biliary sludge and gallstones in pregnancy: incidence, risk factors, and natural history.* Ann Intern Med, 1993. **119**(2): p. 116-20.

35. Chiu, K.C., et al., *Insulin sensitivity is inversely correlated with plasma intact parathyroid hormone level.* Metabolism, 2000. **49**(11): p. 1501-5.

36. Saxe, A.W., et al., *Parathyroid hormone decreases in vivo insulin effect on glucose utilization.* Calcif Tissue Int, 1995. **57**(2): p. 127-32.

37. Kurella, M., J.C. Lo, and G.M. Chertow, *Metabolic syndrome and the risk for chronic kidney disease among nondiabetic adults.* J Am Soc Nephrol, 2005. **16**(7): p. 2134-40.

38. Chen, J., et al., *Insulin resistance and risk of chronic kidney disease in nondiabetic US adults.* J Am Soc Nephrol, 2003. **14**(2): p. 469-77.

39. Cusumano, A.M., et al., *Glomerular hypertrophy is associated with hyperinsulinemia and precedes overt diabetes in aging rhesus monkeys.* Am J Kidney Dis, 2002. **40**(5): p. 1075-85.

Chapter 8

1. GBD 2017 Diet Collaborators, *Health effects of dietary risks in 195 countries, 1990-2017: a systematic analysis for the Global Burden of Disease Study 2017.* Lancet, 2019. **393**(10184): 1958-72.

2. Carlsson, S., et al., *Weight history, glucose intolerance, and insulin levels in middle-aged Swedish men.* Am J Epidemiol, 1998. **148**(6): p. 539-45.

3. Bao, W., S.R. Srinivasan, and G.S. Berenson, *Persistent elevation of plasma insulin levels is associated with increased cardiovascular risk in children and young adults. The Bogalusa Heart Study.* Circulation, 1996. **93**(1): p. 54-9.

4. Lazarus, R., Sparrow, D., et al., *Temporal relations between obesity and insulin: longitudinal data from the Normative Aging Study.* Am J Epidemiol, 1998; **147**: p. 173-179.

5. Hivert, M.F., et al., *The entero-insular axis and adipose tissue-related factors in the prediction of weight gain in humans.* Int J Obesity, 2007; **31**: p. 731-742.

6. Falta, W., *Endocrine Diseases, Including Their Diagnosis and Treatment.* Philadelphia, PA: P. Blakiston's Son & Co., 1923.

7. Zhao, A.Z., K.E. Bornfeldt, and J.A. Beavo, *Leptin inhibits insulin secretion by activation of phosphodiesterase 3B.* J Clin Invest, 1998. **102**(5): p. 869-73.

8. Martin, S.S., A. Qasim, and M.P. Reilly, *Leptin resistance: a possible interface of inflammation and metabolism in obesity-related cardiovascular disease.* J Am Coll Cardiol, 2008. **52**(15): p. 1201-10; Feinstein, A.R., *The treatment of obesity: an analysis of methods, results, and factors which influence success.* J Chronic Dis, 1960. **11**: p. 349-93.

9. Larranaga, A., M.F. Docet, and R.V. Garcia-Mayor, *Disordered eating behaviors in type 1 diabetic patients.* World J Diabetes, 2011. **2**(11): p. 189-95.

10. ADVANCE Collaborative Group, et al., *Intensive blood glucose control and vascular outcomes in patients with type 2 diabetes.* N Engl J Med, 2008. **358**(24): p. 2560-72.

11. Henry, R.R., et al., *Intensive conventional insulin therapy for type II diabetes. Metabolic effects during a 6-mo outpatient trial.* Diabetes Care, 1993. **16**(1): p. 21-31.

12. Torbay, N., et al., *Insulin increases body fat despite control of food intake and physical activity.* Am J Physiol, 1985. **248**(1 Pt 2): p. R120-4.

Chapter 9

1. Pankow, J.S., et al., *Insulin resistance and cardiovascular disease risk factors in children of parents with the insulin resistance (metabolic) syndrome.* Diabetes Care, 2004. **27**(3): p. 775-80.

2. Vaag, A., et al., *Insulin secretion, insulin action, and hepatic glucose production in identical twins discordant for non-insulin-dependent diabetes mellitus.* J Clin Invest, 1995. **95**(2): p. 690-8; Edwards, K.L., et al., *Heritability of factors of the insulin resistance syndrome in women twins.* Genet Epidemiol, 1997. **14**(3): p. 241-53; Mayer, E.J., et al., *Genetic and environmental influences on insulin levels and the insulin resistance syndrome: an analysis of women twins.* Am J Epidemiol, 1996. **143**(4): p. 323-32.

3. Gerich, J.E., *The genetic basis of type 2 diabetes mellitus: impaired insulin secretion versus impaired insulin sensitivity.* Endocr Rev, 1998. **19**(4): p. 491-503.

4. Chiu, K.C., et al., *Insulin sensitivity differs among ethnic groups with a compensatory response in beta-cell function.* Diabetes Care, 2000. **23**(9): p. 1353-8.

5. Fagot-Campagna, A., *Emergence of type 2 diabetes mellitus in children: epidemiological evidence.* J Pediatr Endocrinol Metab, 2000. **13 Suppl 6**: p. 1395-402.

6. Neel, J.V., *Diabetes mellitus: a "thrifty" genotype rendered detrimental by "progress"?* Am J Hum Genet, 1962. **14**: p. 353-62.

7. Baschetti, R., *Diabetes epidemic in newly Westernized populations: is it due to thrifty genes or to genetically unknown foods?* J R Soc Med, 1998. **91**(12): p. 622-5.

8. Fink, R.I., et al., *Mechanisms of insulin resistance in aging.* J Clin Invest, 1983. **71**(6): p. 1523-35.

9. Thurston, R.C., et al., *Vasomotor symptoms and insulin resistance in the study of women's health across the nation.* J Clin Endocrinol Metab, 2012. **97**(10): p. 3487-94.

10. Verma, N., et al., *Growth and hormonal profile from birth to adolescence of a girl with aromatase deficiency.* J Pediatr Endocrinol Metab, 2012. **25**(11-12): p. 1185-90; Rochira, V., et al., *Oestradiol replacement treatment and glucose homeostasis in two men with congenital aromatase deficiency: evidence for a role of oestradiol and sex steroids imbalance on insulin sensitivity in men.* Diabet Med, 2007. **24**(12): p. 1491-5.

11. Carr, M.C., *The emergence of the metabolic syndrome with menopause.* J Clin Endocrinol Metab, 2003. **88**(6): p. 2404-11.

12. Salpeter, S.R., et al., *Meta-analysis: effect of hormone-replacement therapy on components of the metabolic syndrome in postmenopausal women.* Diabetes Obes Metab, 2006. **8**(5): p. 538-54.

13. Muller, M., et al., *Endogenous sex hormones and metabolic syndrome in aging men.* J Clin Endocrinol Metab, 2005. **90**(5): p. 2618-23.

14. Kapoor, D., et al., *Testosterone replacement therapy improves insulin resistance, glycaemic control, visceral adiposity and hypercholesterolaemia in hypogonadal men with type 2 diabetes.* Eur J Endocrinol, 2006. **154**(6): p. 899-906.

Chapter 10

1. Marchesini, G., et al., *Association of nonalcoholic fatty liver disease with insulin resistance.* Am J Med, 1999. **107**(5): p. 450-5.

2. Pontiroli, A.E., M. Alberetto, and G. Pozza, *Patients with insulinoma show insulin resistance in the absence of arterial hypertension.* Diabetologia, 1992. **35**(3): p. 294-5; Pontiroli, A.E., et al., *The glucose clamp technique for the study of patients with hypoglycemia: insulin resistance as a feature of insulinoma.* J Endocrinol Invest, 1990. **13**(3): p. 241-5.

3. Penicaud, L., et al., *Development of VMH obesity: in vivo insulin secretion and tissue insulin sensitivity.* Am J Physiol, 1989. **257**(2 Pt 1): p. E255-60.

4. Del Prato, S., et al., *Effect of sustained physiologic hyperinsulinaemia and hyperglycaemia on insulin secretion and insulin sensitivity in man.* Diabetologia, 1994. **37**(10): p. 1025-35.

5. Henry, R.R., et al., *Intensive conventional insulin therapy for type II diabetes. Metabolic effects during a 6-mo outpatient trial.* Diabetes Care, 1993. **16**(1): p. 21-31.

6. Fourlanos, S., et al., *Insulin resistance is a risk factor for progression to type 1 diabetes.* Diabetologia, 2004. **47**(10): p. 1661-7.

7. Kasper, J.S. and E. Giovannucci, *A meta-analysis of diabetes mellitus and the risk of prostate cancer.* Cancer Epidemiol Biomarkers Prev, 2006. **15**(11): p. 2056-62; Shanik, M.H., et al., *Insulin resistance and hyperinsulinemia: is hyperinsulinemia the cart or the horse?* Diabetes Care, 2008. **31 Suppl 2**: p. S262-8.

8. Gleason, C.E., et al., *Determinants of glucose toxicity and its reversibility in the pancreatic islet beta-cell line, HIT-T15.* Am J Physiol Endocrinol Metab, 2000. **279**(5): p. E997-1002.

9. Lim, E.L., et al., *Reversal of type 2 diabetes: normalisation of beta cell function in association with decreased pancreas and liver triacylglycerol.* Diabetologia, 2011. **54**(10): p. 2506-14.

10. Fiaschi-Taesch, N., et al., *Survey of the human pancreatic beta-cell G1/S proteome reveals a potential therapeutic role for cdk-6 and cyclin D1 in enhancing human beta-cell replication and function in vivo.* Diabetes, 2009. **58**(4): p. 882-93.

11. McFarlane, S.I., et al., *Near-normoglycaemic remission in African-Americans with type 2 diabetes mellitus is associated with recovery of beta cell function.* Diabet Med, 2001. **18**(1): p. 10-6.

12. Meier, J.J., *Beta cell mass in diabetes: a realistic therapeutic target?* Diabetologia, 2008. **51**(5): p. 703-13.

13. Deibert, D.C. and R.A. DeFronzo, *Epinephrine-induced insulin resistance in man.* J Clin Invest, 1980. **65**(3): p. 717-21.

14. Holland, W.L., et al., *Inhibition of ceramide synthesis ameliorates glucocorticoid-, saturated-fat-, and obesity-induced insulin resistance.* Cell Metab, 2007. **5**(3): p. 167-79.

15. Fukuta, H., et al., *Characterization and comparison of insulin resistance induced by Cushing syndrome or diestrus against healthy control dogs as determined by euglycemic-hyperinsulinemic glucose clamp profile glucose infusion rate using an artificial pancreas apparatus.* J Vet Med Sci, 2012. **74**(11): p. 1527-30.

16. Galitzky, J. and A. Bouloumie, *Human visceral-fat-specific glucocorticoid tuning of adipogenesis.* Cell Metab, 2013. **18**(1): p. 3-5.

17. Bastemir, M., et al., *Obesity is associated with increased serum TSH level, independent of thyroid function.* Swiss Med Wkly, 2007. **137**(29-30): p. 431-4.

18. Reinehr, T. and W. Andler, *Thyroid hormones before and after weight loss in obesity.* Arch Dis Child, 2002. **87**(4): p. 320-3.

19. Dimitriadis, G., et al., *The effects of insulin on transport and metabolism of glucose in skeletal muscle from hyperthyroid and hypothyroid rats.* Eur J Clin Invest, 1997. **27**(6): p. 475-83; Dimitriadis, G., et al., *Insulin action in adipose tissue and muscle in hypothyroidism.* J Clin Endocrinol Metab, 2006. **91**(12): p. 4930-7.

20. Arner, P., et al., *Influence of thyroid hormone level on insulin action in human adipose tissue.* Diabetes, 1984. **33**(4): p. 369-75.

Chapter 11

1. Item, F. and D. Konrad, *Visceral fat and metabolic inflammation: the portal theory revisited.* Obes Rev, 2012. **13 Suppl 2**: p. 30-9.

2. Tran, T.T., et al., *Beneficial effects of subcutaneous fat transplantation on metabolism.* Cell Metab, 2008. **7**(5): p. 410-20.

3. Amatruda, J.M., J.N. Livingston, and D.H. Lockwood, *Insulin receptor: role in the resistance of human obesity to insulin.* Science, 1975. **188**(4185): p. 264-6.

4. Taylor, R. and R.R. Holman, *Normal weight individuals who develop Type 2 diabetes: the personal fat threshold.* Clin Sci, 2015. **128**: p. 405-410.

5. Tang, W., et al., *Thiazolidinediones regulate adipose lineage dynamics.* Cell Metab, 2011. **14**(1): p. 116-22.

6. Tandon, P., R. Wafer, and J.E.N. Minchin, *Adipose morphology and metabolic disease.* J Exp Biol, 2018. **221**(Pt Suppl 1).

7. Kim, J.Y., et al., *Adipose tissue insulin resistance in youth on the spectrum from normal weight to obese and from normal glucose tolerance to impaired glucose tolerance to type 2 diabetes.* Diabetes Care, 2019. **42**(2): p. 265-72.

8. Elrayess, M.A., et al., *4-hydroxynonenal causes impairment of human subcutaneous adipogenesis and induction of adipocyte insulin resistance.* Free Radic Biol Med, 2017. **104**: p. 129-37.

9. Prabhu, H.R., *Lipid peroxidation in culinary oils subjected to thermal stress.* Indian J Clin Biochem, 2000. **15**(1): p. 1-5; Schneider, C., et al., *Two distinct pathways of formation of 4-hydroxynonenal. Mechanisms of nonenzymatic transformation of the 9- and 13-hydroperoxides of linoleic acid to 4-hydroxyalkenals.* J Biol Chem, 2001. **276**(24): p. 20831-8; Schneider, C., N.A. Porter, and A.R. Brash, *Routes to 4-hydroxynonenal: fundamental issues in the mechanisms of lipid peroxidation.* J Biol Chem, 2008. **283**(23): p. 15539-43.

10. Guyenet, S.J. and S.E. Carlson, *Increase in adipose tissue linoleic acid of US adults in the last half century.* Adv Nutr, 2015. **6**(6): p. 660-4.

11. Ordonez, M., et al., *Regulation of adipogenesis by ceramide 1-phosphate.* Exp Cell Res, 2018. **372**(2): p. 150-7; Long, S.D. and P.H. Pekala, *Lipid mediators of insulin resistance: ceramide signalling down-regulates GLUT4 gene transcription in 3T3-L1 adipocytes.* Biochem J, 1996. **319 (Pt 1)**: p. 179-84.

12. Weyer, C., et al., *Enlarged subcutaneous abdominal adipocyte size, but not obesity itself, predicts type II diabetes independent of insulin resistance.* Diabetologia, 2000. **43**(12): p. 1498-506.

13. Gustafson, B., et al., *Insulin resistance and impaired adipogenesis.* Trends Endocrinol Metab, 2015. **26**(4): p. 193-200.

14. Chavez, J.A. and S.A. Summers, *Lipid oversupply, selective insulin resistance, and lipotoxicity: molecular mechanisms.* Biochim Biophys Acta, 2010. **1801**(3): p. 252-65.
15. Catanzaro, R., et al., *Exploring the metabolic syndrome: Nonalcoholic fatty pancreas disease.* World J Gastroenterol, 2016. **22**(34): p. 7660-75.
16. Wang, C.Y., et al., *Enigmatic ectopic fat: prevalence of nonalcoholic fatty pancreas disease and its associated factors in a Chinese population.* J Am Heart Assoc, 2014. **3**(1): p. e000297; Lim, E.L., et al., *Reversal of type 2 diabetes: normalisation of beta cell function in association with decreased pancreas and liver triacylglycerol.* Diabetologia, 2011. **54**(10): p. 2506-14.
17. Dube, J.J., et al., *Exercise-induced alterations in intramyocellular lipids and insulin resistance: the athlete's paradox revisited.* Am J Physiol Endocrinol Metab, 2008. **294**(5): p. E882-8.
18. Turner, M.C., Martin, N.R.W., Player, D.J., et al., *Characterising hyperinsulinaemia induced insulin resistance in human skeletal muscle cells.* J Mol Endocrinol, 2020. doi: 10.1530/JME-19-0169.; Hansen, M.E., Tippetts, T.S., et al., *Insulin increases ceramide synthesis in skeletal muscle.* J Diabetes Res, 2014. 765784.
19. Bindlish, S., L.S. Presswala, and F. Schwartz, *Lipodystrophy: Syndrome of severe insulin resistance.* Postgrad Med, 2015. **127**(5): p. 511-6.

Chapter 12

1. Sherrill, J.W. and R. Lawrence, Jr., *Insulin resistance. The mechanisms involved and the influence of infection and refrigeration.* U S Armed Forces Med J, 1950. **1**(12): p. 1399-1409.
2. Drobny, E.C., E.C. Abramson, and G. Baumann, *Insulin receptors in acute infection: a study of factors conferring insulin resistance.* J Clin Endocrinol Metab, 1984. **58**(4): p. 710-6.
3. Chee, B., B. Park, and P.M. Bartold, *Periodontitis and type II diabetes: a two-way relationship.* Int J Evid Based Healthc, 2013. **11**(4): p. 317-29; Taylor, G.W., et al., *Severe periodontitis and risk for poor glycemic control in patients with non-insulin-dependent diabetes mellitus.* J Periodontol, 1996. **67**(10 Suppl): p. 1085-93; Preshaw, P.M., et al., *Periodontitis and diabetes: a two-way relationship.* Diabetologia, 2012. **55**(1): p. 21-31.
4. Liefmann, R., *Endocrine imbalance in rheumatoid arthritis and rheumatoid spondylitis; hyperglycemia unresponsiveness, insulin resistance, increased gluconeogenesis and mesenchymal tissue degeneration; preliminary report.* Acta Med Scand, 1949. **136**(3): p. 226-32; Chung, C.P., et al., *Inflammation-associated insulin resistance: differential effects in rheumatoid arthritis and systemic lupus erythematosus define potential mechanisms.* Arthritis Rheum, 2008. **58**(7): p. 2105-12.
5. Bregenzer, N., et al., *Increased insulin resistance and beta cell activity in patients with Crohn's disease.* Inflamm Bowel Dis, 2006. **12**(1): p. 53-6.
6. Wolfe, R.R., *Substrate utilization/insulin resistance in sepsis/trauma.* Baillieres Clin Endocrinol Metab, 1997. **11**(4): p. 645-57.
7. Visser, M., et al., *Elevated C-reactive protein levels in overweight and obese adults.* JAMA, 1999. **282**(22): p. 2131-5.
8. Hotamisligil, G.S., et al., *IRS-1-mediated inhibition of insulin receptor tyrosine kinase activity in TNF-alpha- and obesity-induced insulin resistance.* Science, 1996. **271**(5249): p. 665-8.

9. Hotamisligil, G.S., N.S. Shargill, and B.M. Spiegelman, *Adipose expression of tumor necrosis factor-alpha: direct role in obesity-linked insulin resistance.* Science, 1993. **259**(5091): p. 87-91.

10. Holland, W.L., et al., *Lipid-induced insulin resistance mediated by the proinflammatory receptor TLR4 requires saturated fatty acid-induced ceramide biosynthesis in mice.* J Clin Invest, 2011. **121**(5): p. 1858-70; Hansen, M.E., et al., *Lipopolysaccharide Disrupts Mitochondrial Physiology in Skeletal Muscle via Disparate Effects on Sphingolipid Metabolism.* Shock, 2015. **44**(6): p. 585-92.

11. Bikman, B.T., *A role for sphingolipids in the pathophysiology of obesity-induced inflammation.* Cell Mol Life Sci, 2012. **69**(13): p. 2135-46.

12. Ibrahim, M.M., *Subcutaneous and visceral adipose tissue: structural and functional differences.* Obes Rev, 2010. **11**(1): p. 11-8.

13. Robinson, A.B., et al., *RAGE signaling by alveolar macrophages influences tobacco smoke-induced inflammation.* Am J Physiol Lung Cell Mol Physiol, 2012. **302**(11): p. L1192-9; Reynolds, P.R., K.M. Wasley, and C.H. Allison, *Diesel particulate matter induces receptor for advanced glycation end-products (RAGE) expression in pulmonary epithelial cells, and RAGE signaling influences NF-kappaB-mediated inflammation.* Environ Health Perspect, 2011. **119**(3): p. 332-6.

14. Chuang, K.J., et al., *The effect of urban air pollution on inflammation, oxidative stress, coagulation, and autonomic dysfunction in young adults.* Am J Respir Crit Care Med, 2007. **176**(4): p. 370-6.

15. Al-Shawwa, B.A., et al., *Asthma and insulin resistance in morbidly obese children and adolescents.* J Asthma, 2007. **44**(6): p. 469-73.

16. Thuesen, B.H., et al., *Insulin resistance as a predictor of incident asthma-like symptoms in adults.* Clin Exp Allergy, 2009. **39**(5): p. 700-7.

17. Shoelson, S.E., L. Herrero, and A. Naaz, *Obesity, inflammation, and insulin resistance.* Gastroenterology, 2007. **132**(6): p. 2169-80.

18. Fisher-Wellman, K.H. and P.D. Neufer, *Linking mitochondrial bioenergetics to insulin resistance via redox biology.* Trends Endocrinol Metab, 2012. **23**(3): p. 142-53.

19. Furukawa, S., et al., *Increased oxidative stress in obesity and its impact on metabolic syndrome.* J Clin Invest, 2004. **114**(12): p. 1752-61; De Mattia, G., et al., *Influence of reduced glutathione infusion on glucose metabolism in patients with non-insulin-dependent diabetes mellitus.* Metabolism, 1998. **47**(8): p. 993-7.

20. Evans, J.L., et al., *Are oxidative stress-activated signaling pathways mediators of insulin resistance and beta-cell dysfunction?* Diabetes, 2003. **52**(1): p. 1-8.

21. Asemi, Z., et al., *Vitamin D supplementation affects serum high-sensitivity C-reactive protein, insulin resistance, and biomarkers of oxidative stress in pregnant women.* J Nutr, 2013. **143**(9): p. 1432-8; Fang, F., Z. Kang, and C. Wong, *Vitamin E tocotrienols improve insulin sensitivity through activating peroxisome proliferator-activated receptors.* Mol Nutr Food Res, 2010. **54**(3): p. 345-52.

22. de Oliveira, A.M., et al., *The effects of lipoic acid and alpha-tocopherol supplementation on the lipid profile and insulin sensitivity of patients with type 2 diabetes mellitus: a randomized, double-blind, placebo-controlled trial.* Diabetes Res Clin Pract, 2011. **92**(2): p. 253-60; Hsu, C.H., et al., *Does supplementation with green tea extract improve insulin resistance in obese type 2 diabetics? A randomized, double-blind, and placebo-controlled clinical trial.* Altern Med Rev, 2011. **16**(2): p. 157-63.

Chapter 13

1. Coogan, P.F., et al., *Air pollution and incidence of hypertension and diabetes mellitus in black women living in Los Angeles.* Circulation, 2012. **125**(6): p. 767-72; Brook, R.D., et al., *Reduced metabolic insulin sensitivity following sub-acute exposures to low levels of ambient fine particulate matter air pollution.* Sci Total Environ, 2013. **448**: p. 66-71.

2. Nemmar, A., et al., *Passage of inhaled particles into the blood circulation in humans.* Circulation, 2002. **105**(4): p. 411-4.

3. Pirkle, J.L., et al., *Exposure of the US population to environmental tobacco smoke: the Third National Health and Nutrition Examination Survey, 1988 to 1991.* JAMA, 1996. **275**(16): p. 1233-40; Pirkle, J.L., et al., *Trends in the exposure of nonsmokers in the U.S. population to secondhand smoke: 1988-2002.* Environ Health Perspect, 2006. **114**(6): p. 853-8.

4. *Vital signs: nonsmokers' exposure to secondhand smoke—United States, 1999-2008.* MMWR Morb Mortal Wkly Rep, 2010. **59**(35): p. 1141-6.

5. Facchini, F.S., et al., *Insulin resistance and cigarette smoking.* Lancet, 1992. **339**(8802): p. 1128-30.

6. Ebersbach-Silva, P., et al., *Cigarette smoke exposure severely reduces peripheral insulin sensitivity without changing GLUT4 expression in oxidative muscle of Wistar rats.* Arq Bras Endocrinol Metabol, 2013. **57**(1): p. 19-26; Thatcher, M.O., et al., *Ceramides mediate cigarette smoke-induced metabolic disruption in mice.* Am J Physiol Endocrinol Metab, 2014. **307**(10): p. E919-27; Borissova, A.M., et al., *The effect of smoking on peripheral insulin sensitivity and plasma endothelin level.* Diabetes Metab, 2004. **30**(2): p. 147-52; Attvall, S., et al., *Smoking induces insulin resistance—a potential link with the insulin resistance syndrome.* J Intern Med, 1993. **233**(4): p. 327-32.

7. Borissova, A.M., et al., *The effect of smoking on peripheral insulin sensitivity and plasma endothelin level.* Diabetes Metab, 2004. **30**(2): p. 147-52; *Vital signs: nonsmokers' exposure to secondhand smoke—United States, 1999-2008.* MMWR Morb Mortal Wkly Rep, 2010. **59**(35): p. 1141-6.

8. Attvall, S., et al., *Smoking induces insulin resistance—a potential link with the insulin resistance syndrome.* J Intern Med, 1993. **233**(4): p. 327-32; Thatcher, M.O., et al., *Ceramides mediate cigarette smoke-induced metabolic disruption in mice.* Am J Physiol Endocrinol Metab, 2014. **307**(10): p. E919-27.

9. Adhami, N., et al., *A Health Threat to Bystanders Living in the Homes of Smokers: How Smoke Toxins Deposited on Surfaces Can Cause Insulin Resistance.* PLoS One, 2016. **11**(3): p. e0149510.

10. Wu, Y., et al., *Activation of AMPKα2 in adipocytes is essential for nicotine-induced insulin resistance in vivo.* Nat Med, 2015. **21**(4): p. 373-82.

11. Bergman, B.C., et al., *Novel and reversible mechanisms of smoking-induced insulin resistance in humans.* Diabetes, 2012. **61**(12): p. 3156-66.

12. Assali, A.R., et al., *Weight gain and insulin resistance during nicotine replacement therapy.* Clin Cardiol, 1999. **22**(5): p. 357-60.

13. van Zyl-Smit, R.N., *Electronic cigarettes: the potential risks outweigh the benefits.* S Afr Med J, 2013. **103**(11): p. 833.

14. Olney, J.W., *Brain lesions, obesity, and other disturbances in mice treated with monosodium glutamate.* Science, 1969. **164**(3880): p. 719-21.

15. Chevassus, H., et al., *Effects of oral monosodium (L)-glutamate on insulin secretion and glucose tolerance in healthy volunteers.* Br J Clin Pharmacol, 2002. **53**(6): p. 641-3.

16. Insawang, T., et al., *Monosodium glutamate (MSG) intake is associated with the prevalence of metabolic syndrome in a rural Thai population.* Nutr Metab (Lond), 2012. **9**(1): p. 50.

17. Cotrim, H.P., et al., *Nonalcoholic fatty liver and insulin resistance among petrochemical workers.* JAMA, 2005. **294**(13): p. 1618-20.

18. Lin, Y., et al., *Exposure to bisphenol A induces dysfunction of insulin secretion and apoptosis through the damage of mitochondria in rat insulinoma (INS-1) cells.* Cell Death Dis, 2013. **4**: p. e460; Magliano, D.J. and J.G. Lyons, *Bisphenol A and diabetes, insulin resistance, cardiovascular disease and obesity: controversy in a (plastic) cup?* J Clin Endocrinol Metab, 2013. **98**(2): p. 502-4.

19. Alonso-Magdalena, P., et al., *Pancreatic insulin content regulation by the estrogen receptor ER alpha.* PLoS One, 2008. **3**(4): p. e2069.

20. Alonso-Magdalena, P., et al., *The estrogenic effect of bisphenol A disrupts pancreatic beta-cell function in vivo and induces insulin resistance.* Environ Health Perspect, 2006. **114**(1): p. 106-12.

21. Lee, D.H., et al., *Low dose organochlorine pesticides and polychlorinated biphenyls predict obesity, dyslipidemia, and insulin resistance among people free of diabetes.* PLoS One, 2011. **6**(1): p. e15977.

22. Kim, K.S., et al., *Associations of organochlorine pesticides and polychlorinated biphenyls in visceral vs. subcutaneous adipose tissue with type 2 diabetes and insulin resistance.* Chemosphere, 2014. **94**: p. 151-7; Lee, D.H., et al., *Association between serum concentrations of persistent organic pollutants and insulin resistance among nondiabetic adults: results from the National Health and Nutrition Examination Survey 1999-2002.* Diabetes Care, 2007. **30**(3): p. 622-8.

23. Kim, K.S., et al., *Associations of organochlorine pesticides and polychlorinated biphenyls in visceral vs. subcutaneous adipose tissue with type 2 diabetes and insulin resistance.* Chemosphere, 2014. **94**: p. 151-7.

24. Melanson, K.J., et al., *Effects of high-fructose corn syrup and sucrose consumption on circulating glucose, insulin, leptin, and ghrelin and on appetite in normal-weight women.* Nutrition, 2007. **23**(2): p. 103-12; Basciano, H., L. Federico, and K. Adeli, *Fructose, insulin resistance, and metabolic dyslipidemia.* Nutr Metab (Lond), 2005. **2**(1): p. 5.

25. Vos, M.B. and C.J. McClain, *Fructose takes a toll.* Hepatology, 2009. **50**(4): p. 1004-6.

26. Diniz, Y.S., et al., *Effects of N-acetylcysteine on sucrose-rich diet-induced hyperglycaemia, dyslipidemia and oxidative stress in rats.* Eur J Pharmacol, 2006. **543**(1-3): p. 151-7; Blouet, C., et al., *Dietary cysteine alleviates sucrose-induced oxidative stress and insulin resistance.* Free Radic Biol Med, 2007. **42**(7): p. 1089-97; Feillet-Coudray, C., et al., *Oxidative stress in rats fed a high-fat high-sucrose diet and preventive effect of polyphenols: Involvement of mitochondrial and NAD(P)H oxidase systems.* Free Radic Biol Med, 2009. **46**(5): p. 624-32.

27. Hu, Y., et al., *Relations of glycemic index and glycemic load with plasma oxidative stress markers.* Am J Clin Nutr, 2006. **84**(1): p. 70-6; quiz 266-7.

28. Nettleton, J.A., et al., *Diet soda intake and risk of incident metabolic syndrome and type 2 diabetes in the Multi-Ethnic Study of Atherosclerosis (MESA).* Diabetes Care, 2009. **32**(4): p. 688-94.

29. Blundell, J.E. and A.J. Hill, *Paradoxical effects of an intense sweetener (aspartame) on appetite.* Lancet, 1986. **1**(8489): p. 1092-3.

30. Swithers, S.E. and T.L. Davidson, *A role for sweet taste: calorie predictive relations in energy regulation by rats.* Behav Neurosci, 2008. **122**(1): p. 161-73.

31. Tonosaki, K., et al., *Relationships between insulin release and taste.* Biomed Res, 2007. **28**(2): p. 79-83.

32. Anton, S.D., et al., *Effects of stevia, aspartame, and sucrose on food intake, satiety, and post-prandial glucose and insulin levels.* Appetite, 2010. **55**(1): p. 37-43.

33. Wolf-Novak, L.C., et al., *Aspartame ingestion with and without carbohydrate in phenyl-ketonuric and normal subjects: effect on plasma concentrations of amino acids, glucose, and insulin.* Metabolism, 1990. **39**(4): p. 391-6.

34. Spiers, P.A., et al., *Aspartame: neuropsychologic and neurophysiologic evaluation of acute and chronic effects.* Am J Clin Nutr, 1998. **68**(3): p. 531-7.

35. Beards, E., K. Tuohy, and G. Gibson, *A human volunteer study to assess the impact of con-fectionery sweeteners on the gut microbiota composition.* Br J Nutr, 2010. **104**(5): p. 701-8.

36. Suez, J., et al., *Artificial sweeteners induce glucose intolerance by altering the gut micro-biota.* Nature, 2014. **514**(7521): p. 181-6.

37. Fageras Bottcher, M., et al., *A TLR4 polymorphism is associated with asthma and reduced lipopolysaccharide-induced interleukin-12(p70) responses in Swedish children.* J Allergy Clin Immunol, 2004. **114**(3): p. 561-7.

38. Ruiz, A.G., et al., *Lipopolysaccharide-binding protein plasma levels and liver TNF-alpha gene expression in obese patients: evidence for the potential role of endotoxin in the pathogen-esis of non-alcoholic steatohepatitis.* Obes Surg, 2007. **17**(10): p. 1374-80.

39. Cani, P.D., et al., *Metabolic endotoxemia initiates obesity and insulin resistance.* Diabetes, 2007. **56**(7): p. 1761-2.

40. Dekker, M.J., et al., *Fructose: a highly lipogenic nutrient implicated in insulin resistance, hepatic steatosis, and the metabolic syndrome.* Am J Physiol Endocrinol Metab, 2010. **299**(5): p. E685-94.

41. Wurfel, M.M., et al., *Lipopolysaccharide (LPS)-binding protein is carried on lipoproteins and acts as a cofactor in the neutralization of LPS.* J Exp Med, 1994. **180**(3): p. 1025-35; Sprong, T., et al., *Human lipoproteins have divergent neutralizing effects on E. coli LPS, N. meningitidis LPS, and complete Gram-negative bacteria.* J Lipid Res, 2004. **45**(4): p. 742-9; Vreugdenhil, A.C., et al., *LPS-binding protein circulates in association with apoB-containing lipoproteins and enhances endotoxin-LDL/VLDL interaction.* J Clin Invest, 2001. **107**(2): p. 225-34; Munford, R.S., J.M. Andersen, and J.M. Dietschy, *Sites of tissue binding and uptake in vivo of bacterial lipopolysaccharide-high density lipoprotein complexes: studies in the rat and squirrel monkey.* J Clin Invest, 1981. **68**(6): p. 1503-13.

42. Shor, R., et al., *Low serum LDL cholesterol levels and the risk of fever, sepsis, and malig-nancy.* Ann Clin Lab Sci, 2007. **37**(4): p. 343-8; Kaysen, G.A., et al., *Lipid levels are inversely associated with infectious and all-cause mortality: international MONDO study results.* J Lipid Res, 2018. **59**(8): p. 1519-1528.

43. Weder, A.B. and B.M. Egan, *Potential deleterious impact of dietary salt restriction on car-diovascular risk factors.* Klin Wochenschr, 1991. **69 Suppl 25**: p. 45-50.

44. Garg, R., et al., *Low-salt diet increases insulin resistance in healthy subjects.* Metabolism, 2011. **60**(7): p. 965-8.

45. Luther, J.M., *Effects of aldosterone on insulin sensitivity and secretion.* Steroids, 2014. **91**: p. 54-60.

46. He, Y., et al., *The transcriptional repressor DEC2 regulates sleep length in mammals.* Sci-ence, 2009. **325**(5942): p. 866-70.

47. Spiegel, K., R. Leproult, and E. Van Cauter, *Impact of sleep debt on metabolic and endo-crine function.* Lancet, 1999. **354**(9188): p. 1435-9.

48. Sweeney, E.L., et al., *Skeletal muscle insulin signaling and whole-body glucose metabolism following acute sleep restriction in healthy males.* Physiol Rep, 2017. **5**(23).

49. Gil-Lozano, M., et al., *Short-term sleep deprivation with nocturnal light exposure alters time-dependent glucagon-like peptide-1 and insulin secretion in male volunteers.* Am J Physiol Endocrinol Metab, 2016. **310**(1): p. E41-50.

50. Baoying, H., et al., *Association of napping and night-time sleep with impaired glucose regulation, insulin resistance and glycated haemoglobin in Chinese middle-aged adults with no diabetes: a cross-sectional study.* BMJ Open, 2014. **4**(7): p. e004419.

51. Amati, F., et al., *Physical inactivity and obesity underlie the insulin resistance of aging.* Diabetes Care, 2009. **32**(8): p. 1547-9.

52. Hamburg, N.M., et al., *Physical inactivity rapidly induces insulin resistance and microvascular dysfunction in healthy volunteers.* Arterioscler Thromb Vasc Biol, 2007. **27**(12): p. 2650-6; Liatis, S., et al., *Vinegar reduces postprandial hyperglycaemia in patients with type II diabetes when added to a high, but not to a low, glycaemic index meal.* Eur J Clin Nutr, 2010. **64**(7): p. 727-32.

53. Pereira, A.F., et al., *Muscle tissue changes with aging.* Acta Med Port, 2013. **26**(1): p. 51-5.

54. Myllynen, P., V.A. Koivisto, and E.A. Nikkila, *Glucose intolerance and insulin resistance accompany immobilization.* Acta Med Scand, 1987. **222**(1): p. 75-81.

55. Crossland, H., et al., *The impact of immobilisation and inflammation on the regulation of muscle mass and insulin resistance: different routes to similar end-points.* J Physiol, 2019. **597**(5): p. 1259-70.

56. Kwon, O.S., et al., *MyD88 regulates physical inactivity-induced skeletal muscle inflammation, ceramide biosynthesis signaling, and glucose intolerance.* Am J Physiol Endocrinol Metab, 2015. **309**(1): p. E11-21.

57. Yates, T., et al., *Self-reported sitting time and markers of inflammation, insulin resistance, and adiposity.* Am J Prev Med, 2012. **42**(1): p. 1-7.

58. Dunstan, D.W., et al., *Breaking up prolonged sitting reduces postprandial glucose and insulin responses.* Diabetes Care, 2012. **35**(5): p. 976-83.

59. Tabata, I., et al., *Resistance training affects GLUT-4 content in skeletal muscle of humans after 19 days of head-down bed rest.* J Appl Physiol (1985), 1999. **86**(3): p. 909-14.

Chapter 14

1. Bergman, B.C., et al., *Muscle sphingolipids during rest and exercise: a C18:0 signature for insulin resistance in humans.* Diabetologia, 2016. **59**(4): p. 785-98.

2. Hughes, V.A., et al., *Exercise increases muscle GLUT-4 levels and insulin action in subjects with impaired glucose tolerance.* Am J Physiol, 1993. **264**(6 Pt 1): p. E855-62.

3. Lehmann, R., et al., *Loss of abdominal fat and improvement of the cardiovascular risk profile by regular moderate exercise training in patients with NIDDM.* Diabetologia, 1995. **38**(11): p. 1313-9.

4. Oh, S., et al., *Exercise reduces inflammation and oxidative stress in obesity-related liver diseases.* Med Sci Sports Exerc, 2013. **45**(12): p. 2214-22.

5. Kubitz, K.A., et al., *The effects of acute and chronic exercise on sleep. A meta-analytic review.* Sports Med, 1996. **21**(4): p. 277-91; de Geus, E.J., L.J. van Doornen, and J.F. Orlebeke, *Regular exercise and aerobic fitness in relation to psychological make-up and physiological stress reactivity.* Psychosom Med, 1993. **55**(4): p. 347-63; Gerber, M., et al., *Fitness and exercise as correlates of sleep complaints: is it all in our minds?* Med Sci Sports Exerc, 2010. **42**(5): p. 893-901.

6. Miller, W.C., D.M. Koceja, and E.J. Hamilton, *A meta-analysis of the past 25 years of weight loss research using diet, exercise or diet plus exercise intervention.* Int J Obes Relat Metab Disord, 1997. **21**(10): p. 941-7; Kratz, M., T. Baars, and S. Guyenet, *The relationship between high-fat dairy consumption and obesity, cardiovascular, and metabolic disease.* Eur J Nutr, 2013. **52**(1): p. 1-24.

7. Ferguson, M.A., et al., *Effects of exercise training and its cessation on components of the insulin resistance syndrome in obese children.* Int J Obes Relat Metab Disord, 1999. **23**(8): p. 889-95; Poehlman, E.T., et al., *Effects of resistance training and endurance training on insulin sensitivity in nonobese, young women: a controlled randomized trial.* J Clin Endocrinol Metab, 2000. **85**(7): p. 2463-8; Miller, J.P., et al., *Strength training increases insulin action in healthy 50- to 65-yr-old men.* J Appl Physiol (1985), 1994. **77**(3): p. 1122-7.

8. Ishii, T., et al., *Resistance training improves insulin sensitivity in NIDDM subjects without altering maximal oxygen uptake.* Diabetes Care, 1998. **21**(8): p. 1353-5; Ibanez, J., et al., *Twice-weekly progressive resistance training decreases abdominal fat and improves insulin sensitivity in older men with type 2 diabetes.* Diabetes Care, 2005. **28**(3): p. 662-7.

9. Eriksson, J., et al., *Aerobic endurance exercise or circuit-type resistance training for individuals with impaired glucose tolerance?* Horm Metab Res, 1998. **30**(1): p. 37-41.

10. Grontved, A., et al., *A prospective study of weight training and risk of type 2 diabetes mellitus in men.* Arch Intern Med, 2012. **172**(17): p. 1306-12.

11. Lee, S., et al., *Effects of aerobic versus resistance exercise without caloric restriction on abdominal fat, intrahepatic lipid, and insulin sensitivity in obese adolescent boys: a randomized, controlled trial.* Diabetes, 2012. **61**(11): p. 2787-95.

12. Yardley, J.E., et al., *Resistance versus aerobic exercise: acute effects on glycemia in type 1 diabetes.* Diabetes Care, 2013. **36**(3): p. 537-42.

13. Kavookjian, J., B.M. Elswick, and T. Whetsel, *Interventions for being active among individuals with diabetes: a systematic review of the literature.* Diabetes Educ, 2007. **33**(6): p. 962-88; discussion 989-90.

14. Taylor, H.L., et al., *Post-exercise carbohydrate-energy replacement attenuates insulin sensitivity and glucose tolerance the following morning in healthy adults.* Nutrients, 2018. **10**(2).

15. Achten, J., M. Gleeson, and A.E. Jeukendrup, *Determination of the exercise intensity that elicits maximal fat oxidation.* Med Sci Sports Exerc, 2002. **34**(1): p. 92-7.

16. Babraj, J.A., et al., *Extremely short duration high intensity interval training substantially improves insulin action in young healthy males.* BMC Endocr Disord, 2009. **9**: p. 3.

17. Orava, J., et al., *Different metabolic responses of human brown adipose tissue to activation by cold and insulin.* Cell Metab, 2011. **14**(2): p. 272-9.

18. Iwen, K.A., et al., *Cold-induced brown adipose tissue activity alters plasma fatty acids and improves glucose metabolism in men.* J Clin Endocrinol Metab, 2017. **102**(11): p. 4226-34; Saito, M., et al., *High incidence of metabolically active brown adipose tissue in healthy adult humans: effects of cold exposure and adiposity.* Diabetes, 2009. **58**(7): p. 1526-31.

19. Sasaki, Y. and H. Takahashi, *Insulin secretion in sheep exposed to cold.* J Physiol, 1980. **306**: p. 323-35; Harada, E., Y. Habara, and T. Kanno, *Cold acclimation in insulin secretion of isolated perfused pancreas of the rat.* Am J Physiol, 1982. **242**(6): p. E360-7.

20. Imbeault, P., I. Depault, and F. Haman, *Cold exposure increases adiponectin levels in men.* Metabolism, 2009. **58**(4): p. 552-9.

Chapter 15

1. Donnelly, J.E., et al., *Effects of a very-low-calorie diet and physical-training regimens on body composition and resting metabolic rate in obese females.* Am J Clin Nutr, 1991. **54**(1): p. 56-61; Duska, F., et al., *Effects of acute starvation on insulin resistance in obese patients with and without type 2 diabetes mellitus.* Clin Nutr, 2005. **24**(6): p. 1056-64; Bacon, L., et al., *Low bone mass in premenopausal chronic dieting obese women.* Eur J Clin Nutr, 2004. **58**(6): p. 966-71.

2. Kanis, J.A., et al., *Anorexia nervosa: a clinical, psychiatric, and laboratory study. I. Clinical and laboratory investigation.* Q J Med, 1974. **43**(170): p. 321-38.

3. Koffler, M. and E.S. Kisch, *Starvation diet and very-low-calorie diets may induce insulin resistance and overt diabetes mellitus.* J Diabetes Complications, 1996. **10**(2): p. 109-12.

4. Douyon, L. and D.E. Schteingart, *Effect of obesity and starvation on thyroid hormone, growth hormone, and cortisol secretion.* Endocrinol Metab Clin North Am, 2002. **31**(1): p. 173-89.

5. Maratou, E., et al., *Studies of insulin resistance in patients with clinical and subclinical hypothyroidism.* Eur J Endocrinol, 2009. **160**(5): p. 785-90.

6. Kahleova, H., et al., *Vegetarian diet improves insulin resistance and oxidative stress markers more than conventional diet in subjects with type 2 diabetes.* Diabet Med, 2011. **28**(5): p. 549-59.

7. Barnard, N.D., et al., *The effects of a low-fat, plant-based dietary intervention on body weight, metabolism, and insulin sensitivity.* Am J Med, 2005. **118**(9): p. 991-7.

8. Shukla, A.P., et al., *The impact of food order on postprandial glycaemic excursions in prediabetes.* Diabetes Obes Metab, 2019. **21**(2): p. 377-81.

9. Marshall, J.A., D.H. Bessesen, and R.F. Hamman, *High saturated fat and low starch and fibre are associated with hyperinsulinaemia in a non-diabetic population: the San Luis Valley Diabetes Study.* Diabetologia, 1997. **40**(4): p. 430-8.

10. Tagliaferro, V., et al., *Moderate guar-gum addition to usual diet improves peripheral sensitivity to insulin and lipaemic profile in NIDDM.* Diabete Metab, 1985. **11**(6): p. 380-5.

11. Cavallo-Perin, P., et al., *Dietary guar gum supplementation does not modify insulin resistance in gross obesity.* Acta Diabetol Lat, 1985. **22**(2): p. 139-42.

12. McKeown, N.M., et al., *Carbohydrate nutrition, insulin resistance, and the prevalence of the metabolic syndrome in the Framingham Offspring Cohort.* Diabetes Care, 2004. **27**(2): p. 538-46.

13. Chandalia, M., et al., *Beneficial effects of high dietary fiber intake in patients with type 2 diabetes mellitus.* N Engl J Med, 2000. **342**(19): p. 1392-8.

14. Lunde, M.S., et al., *Variations in postprandial blood glucose responses and satiety after intake of three types of bread.* J Nutr Metab, 2011. **2011**: p. 437587.

15. Frost, G.S., et al., *The effects of fiber enrichment of pasta and fat content on gastric emptying, GLP-1, glucose, and insulin responses to a meal.* Eur J Clin Nutr, 2003. **57**(2): p. 293-8.

16. Weickert, M.O. and A.F. Pfeiffer, *Metabolic effects of dietary fiber consumption and prevention of diabetes.* J Nutr, 2008. **138**(3): p. 439-42.

17. Popkin, B.M. and K.J. Duffey, *Does hunger and satiety drive eating anymore? Increasing eating occasions and decreasing time between eating occasions in the United States.* Am J Clin Nutr, 2010. **91**(5): p. 1342-7.

18. Horne, B.D., et al., *Relation of routine, periodic fasting to risk of diabetes mellitus, and coronary artery disease in patients undergoing coronary angiography.* Am J Cardiol, 2012. **109**(11): p. 1558-62.

19. Hutchison, A.T. and L.K. Heilbronn, *Metabolic impacts of altering meal frequency and timing—Does when we eat matter?* Biochimie, 2016. **124**: p. 187-97; Kahleova, H., et al., *Eating two larger meals a day (breakfast and lunch) is more effective than six smaller meals in a reduced-energy regimen for patients with type 2 diabetes: a randomised crossover study.* Diabetologia, 2014. **57**(8): p. 1552-60.

20. Halberg, N., et al., *Effect of intermittent fasting and refeeding on insulin action in healthy men.* J Appl Physiol (1985), 2005. **99**(6): p. 2128-36.

21. Soeters, M.R., et al., *Intermittent fasting does not affect whole-body glucose, lipid, or protein metabolism.* Am J Clin Nutr, 2009. **90**(5): p. 1244-51.

22. Furmli, S., et al., *Therapeutic use of intermittent fasting for people with type 2 diabetes as an alternative to insulin.* BMJ Case Rep, 2018. **2018**.

23. Zakaria, A., *Ramadan-like fasting reduces carbonyl stress and improves glycemic control in insulin treated type 2 diabetes mellitus patients.* Life Sci J, 2013. **10**(2): p. 384-90.

24. Harvie, M.N., et al., *The effects of intermittent or continuous energy restriction on weight loss and metabolic disease risk markers: a randomized trial in young overweight women.* Int J Obes (Lond), 2011. **35**(5): p. 714-27.

25. McCutcheon, N.B. and A.M. Tennissen, *Hunger and appetitive factors during total parenteral nutrition.* Appetite, 1989. **13**(2): p. 129-41.

26. de Graaf, C., et al., *Short-term effects of different amounts of protein, fats, and carbohydrates on satiety.* Am J Clin Nutr, 1992. **55**(1): p. 33-8.

27. Stewart, W.K. and L.W. Fleming, *Features of a successful therapeutic fast of 382 days' duration.* Postgrad Med J, 1973. **49**(569): p. 203-9.

28. Mehanna, H.M., J. Moledina, and J. Travis, *Refeeding syndrome: what it is, and how to prevent and treat it.* BMJ, 2008. **336**(7659): p. 1495-8.

29. Bolli, G.B., et al., *Demonstration of a dawn phenomenon in normal human volunteers.* Diabetes, 1984. **33**(12): p. 1150-3.

30. Jarrett, R.J., et al., *Diurnal variation in oral glucose tolerance: blood sugar and plasma insulin levels morning, afternoon, and evening.* Br Med J, 1972. **1**(5794): p. 199-201.

31. Schmidt, M.I., et al., *The dawn phenomenon, an early morning glucose rise: implications for diabetic intraday blood glucose variation.* Diabetes Care, 1981. **4**(6): p. 579-85.

32. Schlundt, D.G., et al., *The role of breakfast in the treatment of obesity: a randomized clinical trial.* Am J Clin Nutr, 1992. **55**(3): p. 645-51.

33. Dhurandhar, E.J., et al., *The effectiveness of breakfast recommendations on weight loss: a randomized controlled trial.* Am J Clin Nutr, 2014. **100**(2): p. 507-13.

34. Carrasco-Benso, M.P., et al., *Human adipose tissue expresses intrinsic circadian rhythm in insulin sensitivity.* FASEB J, 2016. **30**(9): p. 3117-23.

35. Chakrabarti, P., et al., *Insulin inhibits lipolysis in adipocytes via the evolutionarily conserved mTORC1-Egr1-ATGL-mediated pathway.* Mol Cell Biol, 2013. **33**(18): p. 3659-66.

36. Stahl, A., et al., *Insulin causes fatty acid transport protein translocation and enhanced fatty acid uptake in adipocytes.* Dev Cell, 2002. **2**(4): p. 477-88.

37. Unger, R.H., *Glucagon and the insulin: glucagon ratio in diabetes and other catabolic illnesses.* Diabetes, 1971. **20**(12): p. 834-8; Muller, W.A., G.R. Faloona, and R.H. Unger, *The effect of alanine on glucagon secretion.* J Clin Invest, 1971. **50**(10): p. 2215-8.

38. Hans-Rudolf Berthoud, R.J.S., *Neural and metabolic control of macronutrient intake.* 1999: CRC Press. 528.

39. Goodman, B.E., *Insights into digestion and absorption of major nutrients in humans.* Adv Physiol Educ, 2010. **34**(2): p. 44-53.

40. Unger, R.H., *Insulin-glucagon ratio.* Isr J Med Sci, 1972. **8**(3): p. 252-7.

41. US Centers for Disease Control and Prevention, *Trends in intake of energy and macronutrients—United States, 1971-2000.* MMWR Morb Mortal Wkly Rep, 2004. **53**(4): p. 80-2.

42. Shai, I., et al., *Weight loss with a low-carbohydrate, Mediterranean, or low-fat diet.* N Engl J Med, 2008. **359**(3): p. 229-41.

43. Volek, J.S., et al., *Dietary carbohydrate restriction induces a unique metabolic state positively affecting atherogenic dyslipidemia, fatty acid partitioning, and metabolic syndrome.* Prog Lipid Res, 2008. **47**(5): p. 307-18.

44. Nielsen, J.V. and E.A. Joensson, *Low-carbohydrate diet in type 2 diabetes: stable improvement of bodyweight and glycemic control during 44 months follow-up.* Nutr Metab (Lond), 2008. **5**: p. 14.

45. Garg, A., S.M. Grundy, and R.H. Unger, *Comparison of effects of high and low carbohydrate diets on plasma lipoproteins and insulin sensitivity in patients with mild NIDDM.* Diabetes, 1992. **41**(10): p. 1278-85.

46. Hu, T., et al., *Effects of low-carbohydrate diets versus low-fat diets on metabolic risk factors: a meta-analysis of randomized controlled clinical trials.* Am J Epidemiol, 2012. **176 Suppl** 7: p. S44-54; Santos, F.L., et al., *Systematic review and meta-analysis of clinical trials of the effects of low carbohydrate diets on cardiovascular risk factors.* Obes Rev, 2012. **13**(11): p. 1048-66.

47. *Lifestyle Management: Standards of Medical Care in Diabetes—2019.* Diabetes Care, 2019. 42(s1): p. S46-S60.

48. Foster-Powell, K., S.H. Holt, and J.C. Brand-Miller, *International table of glycemic index and glycemic load values: 2002.* Am J Clin Nutr, 2002. **76**(1): p. 5-56.

49. Fukagawa, N.K., et al., *High-carbohydrate, high-fiber diets increase peripheral insulin sensitivity in healthy young and old adults.* Am J Clin Nutr, 1990. **52**(3): p. 524-8; Siri-Tarino, P.W., et al., *Saturated fat, carbohydrate, and cardiovascular disease.* Am J Clin Nutr, 2010. **91**(3): p. 502-9.

50. Ebbeling, C.B., et al., *Effects of a low-glycemic load vs low-fat diet in obese young adults: a randomized trial.* JAMA, 2007. **297**(19): p. 2092-102.

51. Smith, U., *Impaired ('diabetic') insulin signaling and action occur in fat cells long before glucose intolerance—is insulin resistance initiated in the adipose tissue?* Int J Obes Relat Metab Disord, 2002. **26**(7): p. 897-904.

52. Gardner, C.D., et al., *Comparison of the Atkins, Zone, Ornish, and LEARN diets for change in weight and related risk factors among overweight premenopausal women: the A TO Z Weight Loss Study: a randomized trial.* JAMA, 2007. **297**(9): p. 969-77; McClain, A.D., et al., *Adherence to a low-fat vs. low-carbohydrate diet differs by insulin resistance status.* Diabetes Obes Metab, 2013. **15**(1): p. 87-90.

53. Zeevi, D., et al., *Personalized nutrition by prediction of glycemic responses.* Cell, 2015. **163**(5): p. 1079-94.

54. Goodpaster, B.H., et al., *Skeletal muscle lipid content and insulin resistance: evidence for a paradox in endurance-trained athletes.* J Clin Endocrinol Metab, 2001. **86**(12): p. 5755-61.

55. Bikman, B.T. and S.A. Summers, *Ceramides as modulators of cellular and whole-body metabolism.* J Clin Invest, 2011. **121**(11): p. 4222-30.

56. Helge, J.W., et al., *Muscle ceramide content is similar after 3 weeks' consumption of fat or carbohydrate diet in a crossover design in patients with type 2 diabetes.* Eur J Appl Physiol, 2012. **112**(3): p. 911-8.

57. Volek, J.S., et al., *Carbohydrate restriction has a more favorable impact on the metabolic syndrome than a low fat diet.* Lipids, 2009. **44**(4): p. 297-309.

58. Teng, K.T., et al., *Palm olein and olive oil cause a higher increase in postprandial lipemia compared with lard but had no effect on plasma glucose, insulin and adipocytokines.* Lipids, 2011. **46**(4): p. 381-8.

59. Ramsden, C.E., et al., *Use of dietary linoleic acid for secondary prevention of coronary heart disease and death: evaluation of recovered data from the Sydney Diet Heart Study and updated meta-analysis.* BMJ, 2013. **346**: p. e8707; Gillman, M.W., et al., *Margarine intake and subsequent coronary heart disease in men.* Epidemiology, 1997. **8**(2): p. 144-9; Ramsden, C.E., et al., *Re-evaluation of the traditional diet-heart hypothesis: analysis of recovered data from Minnesota Coronary Experiment (1968-73).* BMJ, 2016. **353**: p. i1246.

60. Rhee, Y. and A. Brundt, *Flaxseed supplementation improved insulin resistance in obese glucose intolerant people: a randomized crossover design.* Nutr J, 2011. **10**(44): p. 1-7.

61. Milder, J. and M. Patel, *Modulation of oxidative stress and mitochondrial function by the ketogenic diet.* Epilepsy Res, 2012. **100**(3): p. 295-303; Forsythe, C.E., et al., *Comparison of low fat and low carbohydrate diets on circulating fatty acid composition and markers of inflammation.* Lipids, 2008. **43**(1): p. 65-77.

62. Nazarewicz, R.R., et al., *Effect of short-term ketogenic diet on redox status of human blood.* Rejuvenation Res, 2007. **10**(4): p. 435-40; Shimazu, T., et al., *Suppression of oxidative stress by beta-hydroxybutyrate, an endogenous histone deacetylase inhibitor.* Science, 2013. **339**(6116): p. 211-4; Maalouf, M., et al., *Ketones inhibit mitochondrial production of reactive oxygen species production following glutamate excitotoxicity by increasing NADH oxidation.* Neuroscience, 2007. **145**(1): p. 256-64; Kim, D.Y., et al., *Ketone bodies are protective against oxidative stress in neocortical neurons.* J Neurochem, 2007. **101**(5): p. 1316-26; Facchini, F.S., et al., *Hyperinsulinemia: the missing link among oxidative stress and age-related diseases?* Free Radic Biol Med, 2000. **29**(12): p. 1302-6; Krieger-Brauer, H.I. and H. Kather, *Human fat cells possess a plasma membrane-bound H2O2-generating system that is activated by insulin via a mechanism bypassing the receptor kinase.* J Clin Invest, 1992. **89**(3): p. 1006-13; Evans, J.L., B.A. Maddux, and I.D. Goldfine, *The molecular basis for oxidative stress-induced insulin resistance.* Antioxid Redox Signal, 2005. **7**(7-8): p. 1040-52.

63. Youm, Y.H., et al., *The ketone metabolite beta-hydroxybutyrate blocks NLRP3 inflammasome-mediated inflammatory disease.* Nat Med, 2015. **21**(3): p. 263-9.

64. Bough, K.J., et al., *Mitochondrial biogenesis in the anticonvulsant mechanism of the ketogenic diet.* Ann Neurol, 2006. **60**(2): p. 223-35.

65. Kim, D.Y., et al., *Ketone bodies are protective against oxidative stress in neocortical neurons.* J Neurochem, 2007. **101**(5): p. 1316-26; Youm, Y.H., et al., *The ketone metabolite beta-hydroxybutyrate blocks NLRP3 inflammasome-mediated inflammatory disease.* Nat Med, 2015. **21**(3): p. 263-9.

66. Edwards, C., N. Copes, and P.C. Bradshaw, *D-ss-hydroxybutyrate: an anti-aging ketone body.* Oncotarget, 2015. **6**(6): p. 3477-8; Roberts, M.N., et al., *A Ketogenic Diet Extends Longevity and Healthspan in Adult Mice.* Cell Metab, 2018. **27**(5): p. 1156.

67. Parker, B., et al., *Beta-hydroxybutyrate favorably alters muscle cell survival and mitochondrial bioenergetics.* FASEB J, 2017. **31**.

68. Cahill, G.F., Jr., *Fuel metabolism in starvation.* Annu Rev Nutr, 2006. **26**: p. 1-22.

69. Myette-Cote, E., et al., *Prior ingestion of exogenous ketone monoester attenuates the glycaemic response to an oral glucose tolerance test in healthy young individuals.* J Physiol, 2018. **596**(8): p. 1385-95.

70. Benedict F.G. and E.P. Joslin, *A Study of Metabolism in Severe Diabetes.* Washington DC: Carnegie Institution of Washington, 1912.

71. Franssila-Kallunki, A. and L. Groop, *Factors associated with basal metabolic rate in patients with type 2 (non-insulin-dependent) diabetes mellitus.* Diabetologia, 1992. **35**(10): p. 962-6; *Weight gain associated with intensive therapy in the diabetes control and complications trial. The DCCT Research Group.* Diabetes Care, 1988. **11**(7): p. 567-73; Nathan, D.M., et al., *Medical management of hyperglycemia in type 2 diabetes: a consensus algorithm for the initiation and adjustment of therapy: a consensus statement of the American Diabetes Association and the European Association for the Study of Diabetes.* Diabetes Care, 2009. **32**(1): p. 193-203.

72. Srivastava, S., et al., *A ketogenic diet increases brown adipose tissue mitochondrial proteins and UCP1 levels in mice.* IUBMB Life, 2013. **65**(1): p. 58-66; Srivastava, S., et al., *Mitochondrial biogenesis and increased uncoupling protein 1 in brown adipose tissue of mice fed a ketone ester diet.* FASEB J, 2012. **26**(6): p. 2351-62.

73. Brehm, B.J., et al., *A randomized trial comparing a very low carbohydrate diet and a calorie-restricted low fat diet on body weight and cardiovascular risk factors in healthy women.* J Clin Endocrinol Metab, 2003. **88**(4): p. 1617-23.

74. Sharman, M.J., et al., *A ketogenic diet favorably affects serum biomarkers for cardiovascular disease in normal-weight men.* J Nutr, 2002. **132**(7): p. 1879-85.

75. Ebbeling, C.B., et al., *Effects of dietary composition on energy expenditure during weight-loss maintenance.* JAMA, 2012. **307**(24): p. 2627-34.

76. Ebbeling, C.B., et al., *Effects of a low carbohydrate diet on energy expenditure during weight loss maintenance: randomized trial.* BMJ, 2018. **363**: p. k4583; Hall, K.D., et al., *Energy expenditure and body composition changes after an isocaloric ketogenic diet in overweight and obese men.* Am J Clin Nutr, 2016. **104**(2): p. 324-33.

77. Sharman, M.J., et al., *A ketogenic diet favorably affects serum biomarkers for cardiovascular disease in normal-weight men.* J Nutr, 2002. **132**(7): p. 1879-85.

78. Westman, E.C., et al., *Effect of a low-carbohydrate, ketogenic diet program compared to a low-fat diet on fasting lipoprotein subclasses.* Int J Cardiol, 2006. **110**(2): p. 212-6.

79. Garvey, W.T., et al., *Effects of insulin resistance and type 2 diabetes on lipoprotein subclass particle size and concentration determined by nuclear magnetic resonance.* Diabetes, 2003. **52**(2): p. 453-62.

80. Gardner, C.D., et al., *Comparison of the Atkins, Zone, Ornish, and LEARN diets for change in weight and related risk factors among overweight premenopausal women: the A TO Z Weight Loss Study: a randomized trial.* JAMA, 2007. **297**(9): p. 969-77.

81. Mavropoulos, J.C., et al., *The effects of a low-carbohydrate, ketogenic diet on the polycystic ovary syndrome: a pilot study.* Nutr Metab (Lond), 2005. **2**: p. 35.

82. Hamalainen, E.K., et al., *Decrease of serum total and free testosterone during a low-fat high-fibre diet.* J Steroid Biochem, 1983. **18**(3): p. 369-70.

83. Molteni, R., et al., *A high-fat, refined sugar diet reduces hippocampal brain-derived neurotrophic factor, neuronal plasticity, and learning.* Neuroscience, 2002. **112**(4): p. 803-14; Jurdak, N. and R.B. Kanarek, *Sucrose-induced obesity impairs novel object recognition learning in young rats.* Physiol Behav, 2009. **96**(1): p. 1-5.

84. Young, K.W., et al., *A randomized, crossover trial of high-carbohydrate foods in nursing home residents with Alzheimer's disease: associations among intervention response, body mass*

index, and behavioral and cognitive function. J Gerontol A Biol Sci Med Sci, 2005. **60**(8): p. 1039-45.

85. Reger, M.A., et al., *Effects of beta-hydroxybutyrate on cognition in memory-impaired adults.* Neurobiol Aging, 2004. **25**(3): p. 311-4.

86. Bredesen, D.E., *Reversal of cognitive decline: a novel therapeutic program.* Aging (Albany NY), 2014. **6**(9): p. 707-17.

87. Berger, A., *Insulin resistance and reduced brain glucose metabolism in the aetiology of Alzheimer's disease.* J Insulin Resistance, 2016. **1**(1).

88. Vanitallie, T.B., et al., *Treatment of Parkinson disease with diet-induced hyperketonemia: a feasibility study.* Neurology, 2005. **64**(4): p. 728-30.

89. Cheng, B., et al., *Ketogenic diet protects dopaminergic neurons against 6-OHDA neurotoxicity via up-regulating glutathione in a rat model of Parkinson's disease.* Brain Res, 2009. **1286**: p. 25-31.

90. Schnabel, T.G., *An experience with a ketogenic dietary in migraine.* Ann Intern Med, 1928. **2**(4): p. 341-7.

91. Barborka, C.J., *Migraine: results of treatments by ketogenic diet in fifty cases.* JAMA, 1930. **95**(24): p. 1825-8.

92. Di Lorenzo, C., et al., *Diet transiently improves migraine in two twin sisters: possible role of ketogenesis?* Funct Neurol, 2013. **28**(4): p. 305-8.

93. Dexter, J.D., J. Roberts, and J.A. Byer, *The five hour glucose tolerance test and effect of low sucrose diet in migraine.* Headache, 1978. **18**(2): p. 91-4.

94. Austin, G.L., et al., *A very low-carbohydrate diet improves gastroesophageal reflux and its symptoms.* Dig Dis Sci, 2006. **51**(8): p. 1307-12.

95. Yancy, W.S., Jr., D. Provenzale, and E.C. Westman, *Improvement of gastroesophageal reflux disease after initiation of a low-carbohydrate diet: five brief case reports.* Altern Ther Health Med, 2001. **7**(6): p. 120, 116-9.

96. Hermanns-Le, T., A. Scheen, and G.E. Pierard, *Acanthosis nigricans associated with insulin resistance: pathophysiology and management.* Am J Clin Dermatol, 2004. **5**(3): p. 199-203.

97. Paoli, A., et al., *Nutrition and acne: therapeutic potential of ketogenic diets.* Skin Pharmacol Physiol, 2012. **25**(3): p. 111-7.

98. Fomin, D.A., B. McDaniel, and J. Crane, *The promising potential role of ketones in inflammatory dermatologic disease: a new frontier in treatment research.* J Dermatolog Treat, 2017: p. 1-16.

99. Tatar, M., A. Bartke, and A. Antebi, *The endocrine regulation of aging by insulin-like signals.* Science, 2003. **299**(5611): p. 1346-51.

100. Li, Y., L. Liu, and T.O. Tollefsbol, *Glucose restriction can extend normal cell lifespan and impair precancerous cell growth through epigenetic control of hTERT and p16 expression.* FASEB J, 2010. **24**(5): p. 1442-53; Mair, W. and A. Dillin, *Aging and survival: the genetics of life span extension by dietary restriction.* Annu Rev Biochem, 2008. **77**: p. 727-54; Anderson, R.M., et al., *Yeast life-span extension by calorie restriction is independent of NAD fluctuation.* Science, 2003. **302**(5653): p. 2124-6.

101. Yancy, W.S., Jr., et al., *A low-carbohydrate, ketogenic diet versus a low-fat diet to treat obesity and hyperlipidemia: a randomized, controlled trial.* Ann Intern Med, 2004. **140**(10): p. 769-77; Gasior, M., M.A. Rogawski, and A.L. Hartman, *Neuroprotective and disease-modifying effects of the ketogenic diet.* Behav Pharmacol, 2006. **17**(5-6): p. 431-9; Wijsman, C.A., et al., *Familial longevity is marked by enhanced insulin sensitivity.* Aging Cell, 2011. **10**(1): p. 114-21.

Chapter 16

1. Bhatti, J.A., et al., *Self-harm emergencies after bariatric surgery: a population-based cohort study*. JAMA Surg, 2015: p. 1-7.
2. Odom, J., et al., *Behavioral predictors of weight regain after bariatric surgery*. Obes Surg, 2010. **20**(3): p. 349-56.
3. Wickremesekera, K., et al., *Loss of insulin resistance after Roux-en-Y gastric bypass surgery: a time course study*. Obes Surg, 2005. **15**(4): p. 474-81.
4. Zhu, Y., et al., *Evaluation of insulin resistance improvement after laparoscopic sleeve gastrectomy or gastric bypass surgery with HOMA-IR*. Biosci Trends, 2017. **11**(6): p. 675-81.
5. Stefater, M.A., et al., *All bariatric surgeries are not created equal: insights from mechanistic comparisons*. Endocr Rev, 2012. **33**(4): p. 595-622.
6. Saliba, C., et al., *Weight regain after sleeve gastrectomy: a look at the benefits of re-sleeve*. Cureus, 2018. **10**(10): p. e3450.

Chapter 17

1. Johnson, J.L., et al., *Identifying prediabetes using fasting insulin levels*. Endocr Pract, 2010. **16**(1): p. 47-52.
2. Crofts, C., et al., *Identifying hyperinsulinaemia in the absence of impaired glucose tolerance: An examination of the Kraft database*. Diabetes Res Clin Pract, 2016. **118**: p. 50-7.
3. Hayashi, T., Boyko, E.J., Sato, K.K., et al., *Patterns of insulin concentration during the OGTT predict the risk of type 2 diabetes in Japanese Americans*. Diabetes Care, 2013. **36**: p. 1229-1235.
4. Westman, E.C. and M.C. Vernon, *Has carbohydrate-restriction been forgotten as a treatment for diabetes mellitus? A perspective on the ACCORD study design*. Nutr Metab (Lond), 2008. **5**: p. 10.
5. Grontved, A., et al., *A prospective study of weight training and risk of type 2 diabetes mellitus in men*. Arch Intern Med, 2012. **172**(17): p. 1306-12.
6. Segerstrom, A.B., et al., *Impact of exercise intensity and duration on insulin sensitivity in women with T2D*. Eur J Intern Med, 2010. **21**(5): p. 404-8.
7. Ismail, A.D., et al., *The effect of short duration resistance training on insulin sensitivity and muscle adaptations in overweight men*. Exp Physiol, 2019.
8. Walton, C.M., et al., *Improvement in glycemic and lipid profiles in type 2 diabetics with a 90-day ketogenic diet*. J Diabetes Res, 2019. **2019**: p. 8681959.
9. Bolton, R.P., et al., *The role of dietary fiber in satiety, glucose, and insulin: studies with fruit and fruit juice*. Am J Clin Nutr, 1981 34(2): 211-7.
10. Liatis, S., et al., *Vinegar reduces postprandial hyperglycaemia in patients with type II diabetes when added to a high, but not to a low, glycaemic index meal*. Eur J Clin Nutr, 2010. **64**(7): p. 727-32; Johnston, C.S., C.M. Kim, and A.J. Buller, *Vinegar improves insulin sensitivity to a high-carbohydrate meal in subjects with insulin resistance or type 2 diabetes*. Diabetes Care, 2004. **27**(1): p. 281-2.
11. Johnston, C.S., A.M. White, and S.M. Kent, *Preliminary evidence that regular vinegar ingestion favorably influences hemoglobin A1c values in individuals with type 2 diabetes mellitus*. Diabetes Res Clin Pract, 2009. **84**(2): p. e15-7.
12. White, A.M. and C.S. Johnston, *Vinegar ingestion at bedtime moderates waking glucose concentrations in adults with well-controlled type 2 diabetes*. Diabetes Care, 2007. **30**(11): p. 2814-5.

13. Maioli, M., et al., *Sourdough-leavened bread improves postprandial glucose and insulin plasma levels in subjects with impaired glucose tolerance.* Acta Diabetol, 2008. **45**(2): p. 91-6.

14. Lappi, J.S., et al., *Sourdough fermentation of wholemeal wheat bread increases solubility of arabinoxylan and protein and decreases postprandial glucose and insulin responses.* J Cereal Sci, 2010. **51**(1): p. 152-8.

15. Ostman, E.M., H.G. Liljeberg Elmstahl, and I.M. Bjorck, *Inconsistency between glycemic and insulinemic responses to regular and fermented milk products.* Am J Clin Nutr, 2001. **74**(1): p. 96-100.

16. Ostadrahimi, A., et al., *Effect of probiotic fermented milk (kefir) on glycemic control and lipid profile in type 2 diabetic patients: a randomized double-blind placebo-controlled clinical trial.* Iran J Public Health, 2015. **44**(2): p. 228-37.

17. An, S.Y., et al., *Beneficial effects of fresh and fermented kimchi in prediabetic individuals.* Ann Nutr Metab, 2013. **63**(1-2): p. 111-9.

18. Cheon, J.M., D.I. Kim, and K.S. Kim, *Insulin sensitivity improvement of fermented Korean Red Ginseng (Panax ginseng) mediated by insulin resistance hallmarks in old-aged ob/ob mice.* J Ginseng Res, 2015. **39**(4): p. 331-7; Kwon, D.Y., et al., *Long-term consumption of fermented soybean-derived Chungkookjang attenuates hepatic insulin resistance in 90% pancreatectomized diabetic rats.* Horm Metab Res, 2007. **39**(10): p. 752-7.

19. Ruan, Y., et al., *Effect of probiotics on glycemic control: a systematic review and meta-analysis of randomized, controlled trials.* PLoS One, 2015. **10**(7): p. e0132121.

20. Morton, R.W., et al., *A systematic review, meta-analysis and meta-regression of the effect of protein supplementation on resistance training-induced gains in muscle mass and strength in healthy adults.* Br J Sports Med, 2018. **52**(6): p. 376-84; Muller, W.A., G.R. Faloona, and R.H. Unger, *The effect of alanine on glucagon secretion.* J Clin Invest, 1971. **50**(10): p. 2215-8; Unger, R.H., *Insulin-glucagon ratio.* Isr J Med Sci, 1972. **8**(3): p. 252-7.

21. Traylor, D.A., S.H.M. Gorissen, and S.M. Phillips, *Perspective: protein requirements and optimal intakes in aging: are we ready to recommend more than the recommended daily allowance?* Adv Nutr, 2018. **9**(3): p. 171-82.

22. Hoffman, J.R. and M.J. Falvo, *Protein—which is best?* J Sports Sci Med, 2004. **3**(3): p. 118-30.

23. Holmberg, S. and A. Thelin, *High dairy fat intake related to less central obesity: a male cohort study with 12 years' follow-up.* Scand J Prim Health Care, 2013. **31**(2): p. 89-94.

24. Yakoob, M.Y., et al., *Circulating biomarkers of dairy fat and risk of incident diabetes mellitus among us men and women in two large prospective cohorts.* Circulation, 2016. **133**(17): p. 1645-54.

25. Humphries, S., H. Kushner, and B. Falkner, *Low dietary magnesium is associated with insulin resistance in a sample of young, nondiabetic Black Americans.* Am J Hypertens, 1999. **12**(8 Pt 1): p. 747-56; Paolisso, G. and E. Ravussin, *Intracellular magnesium and insulin resistance: results in Pima Indians and Caucasians.* J Clin Endocrinol Metab, 1995. **80**(4): p. 1382-5.

26. Paolisso, G., et al., *Daily magnesium supplements improve glucose handling in elderly subjects.* Am J Clin Nutr, 1992. **55**(6): p. 1161-7.

27. Rodriguez-Moran, M. and F. Guerrero-Romero, *Oral magnesium supplementation improves insulin sensitivity and metabolic control in type 2 diabetic subjects: a randomized double-blind controlled trial.* Diabetes Care, 2003. **26**(4): p. 1147-52.

28. Guerrero-Romero, F., et al., *Oral magnesium supplementation improves insulin sensitivity in non-diabetic subjects with insulin resistance. A double-blind placebo-controlled randomized trial.* Diabetes Metab, 2004. **30**(3): p. 253-8.

29. Morris, B.W., et al., *Chromium supplementation improves insulin resistance in patients with type 2 diabetes mellitus.* Diabet Med, 2000. **17**(9): p. 684-5.

30. Blouet, C., et al., *Dietary cysteine alleviates sucrose-induced oxidative stress and insulin resistance.* Free Radic Biol Med, 2007. **42**(7): p. 1089-97.

31. Shalileh, M., et al., *The influence of calcium supplement on body composition, weight loss and insulin resistance in obese adults receiving low calorie diet.* J Res Med Sci, 2010. **15**(4): p. 191-201.

32. Zemel, M.B., et al., *Effects of calcium and dairy on body composition and weight loss in African-American adults.* Obes Res, 2005. **13**(7): p. 1218-25.

33. Zemel, M.B., et al., *Calcium and dairy acceleration of weight and fat loss during energy restriction in obese adults.* Obes Res, 2004. **12**(4): p. 582-90.

34. Pereira, M.A., et al., *Dairy consumption, obesity, and the insulin resistance syndrome in young adults: the CARDIA Study.* JAMA, 2002. **287**(16): p. 2081-9.

35. Chiu, K.C., et al., *Hypovitaminosis D is associated with insulin resistance and beta cell dysfunction.* Am J Clin Nutr, 2004. **79**(5): p. 820-5.

36. von Hurst, P.R., W. Stonehouse, and J. Coad, *Vitamin D supplementation reduces insulin resistance in South Asian women living in New Zealand who are insulin resistant and vitamin D deficient—a randomised, placebo-controlled trial.* Br J Nutr, 2010. **103**(4): p. 549-55.

37. Islam, M.R., *Zinc supplementation for improving glucose handling in pre-diabetes: A double blind randomized placebo controlled pilot study.* Diabetes Res Clin Prac, 2016. **115**: p. 39-46.

38. Roshanravan, N., et al., *Effect of zinc supplementation on insulin resistance, energy and macronutrients intakes in pregnant women with impaired glucose tolerance.* Iran J Public Health, 2015. **44**(2): p. 211-7.

39. Avena, N.M., P. Rada, and B.G. Hoebel, *Evidence for sugar addiction: behavioral and neurochemical effects of intermittent, excessive sugar intake.* Neurosci Biobehav Rev, 2008. **32**(1): p. 20-39.

40. Hutchison, A.T. and L.K. Heilbronn, *Metabolic impacts of altering meal frequency and timing—Does when we eat matter?* Biochimie, 2016. **124**: p. 187-97.

INDEX

ABOUT THE AUTHOR

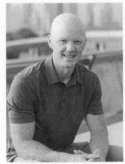

Photo by Leah Aldous

BENJAMIN BIKMAN earned a Ph.D. in Bioenergetics at East Carolina University with a focus on the adaptations to metabolic surgeries in obesity. He continued to explore metabolic disorders, with a particular focus on insulin resistance, as a postdoctoral fellow with the Duke-National University of Singapore Medical School. As a professor at Brigham Young University and the director of its Diabetes Research Lab, Dr. Bikman has continued to study insulin, including its role as a regulator of human metabolism, as well as insulin's relevance in chronic disease. In addition to his research and teaching, Dr. Bikman actively serves as a research mentor to undergraduate and graduate students. He and his students frequently present and publish their findings.

He lives with his family in Provo, Utah.